Sir John's Table

Sir John's TABLE

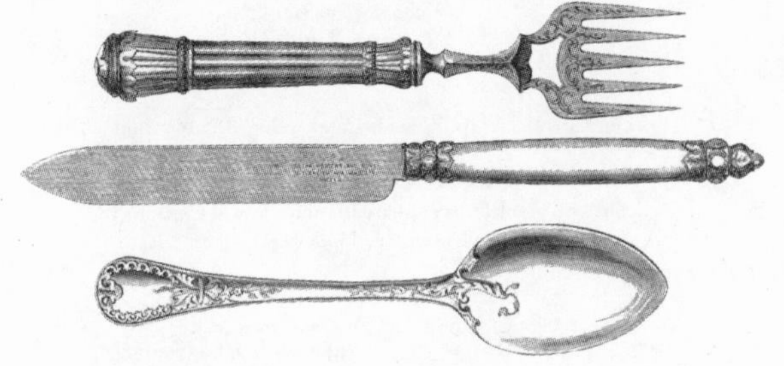

The Culinary Life & Times of Canada's First Prime Minister

LINDY MECHEFSKE

Goose Lane Editions

Edited by Elizabeth Eve.
Cover and page design by Julie Scriver.
Cover illustration (utensils): www.thegraphicsfairy.com.
Printed in Canada.
10 9 8 7 6 5 4 3 2 1

Library and Archives Canada Cataloguing in Publication

Mechefske, Lindy, 1961-, author
Sir John's table : the culinary life and times of Canada's first prime minister / Lindy Mechefske.

Includes bibliographical references and index.
Issued in print and electronic formats.
ISBN 978-0-86492-881-8 (pbk.). -- ISBN 978-0-86492-839-9 (epub).
-- ISBN 978-0-86492-840-5 (mobi)

1. Cooking -- Canada -- History -- 19th century.
2. Macdonald, John A. (John Alexander), 1815-1891.
3. Diet -- Canada -- History -- 19th century.
4. Dinners and dining -- Canada -- History -- 19th century.
5. Food habits -- Canada -- History -- 19th century.
6. Canada -- Social life and customs -- 19th century. I. Title.

TX645.M43 2015 641.50971'09034 C2015-901863-3
C2015-901864-1

We acknowledge the generous support of the Government of Canada, the Canada Council for the Arts, and the Government of New Brunswick.

Nous reconnaissons l'appui généreux du gouvernement du Canada, du Conseil des arts du Canada, et du gouvernement du Nouveau-Brunswick.

Goose Lane Editions
500 Beaverbrook Court, Suite 330
Fredericton, New Brunswick
CANADA E3B 5X4
www.gooselane.com

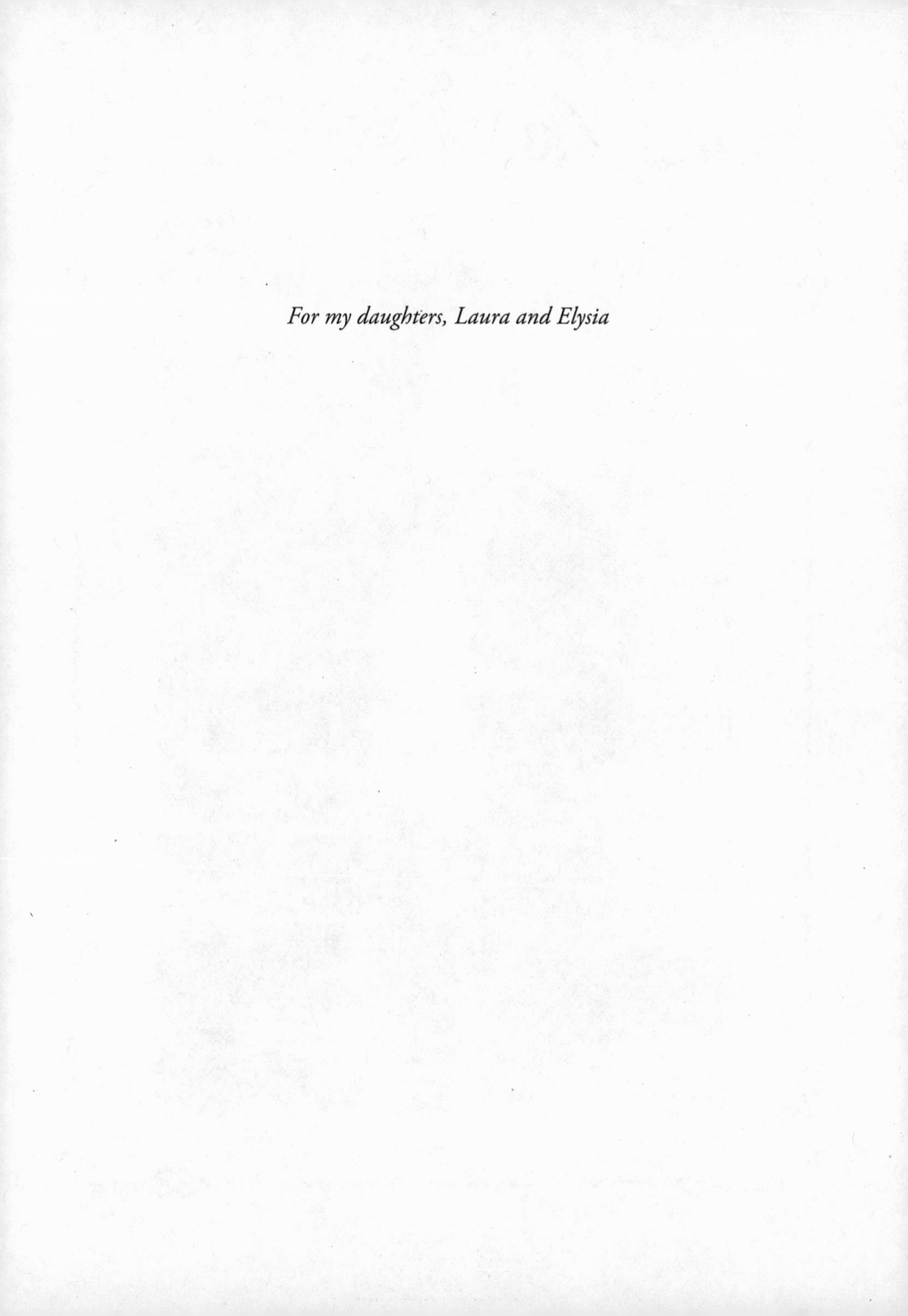

For my daughters, Laura and Elysia

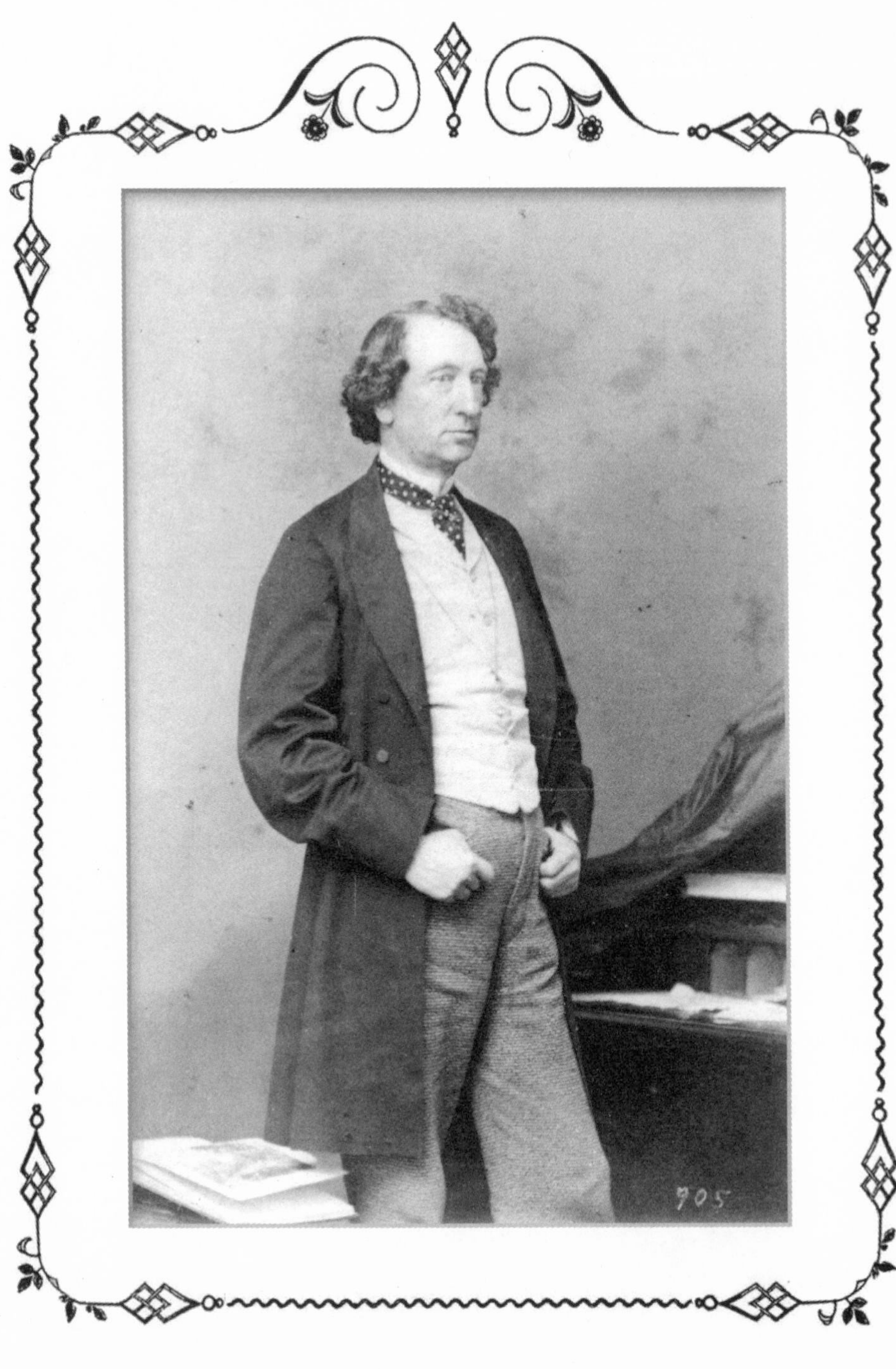

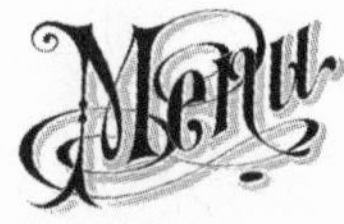

Sir John A. Macdonald Timeline

1815 January 10—official date of birth as listed in the Registry of Births, Scotland, for John A. Macdonald.

1815 January 11—date that Hugh Macdonald, John A. Macdonald's father, records as John A.'s birthdate.

1820 June—Family leaves Glasgow, Scotland, and boards the *Earl of Buckinghamshire* bound for Quebec City.

1820 August 13—Macdonald family arrives at Col. Donald and Anna Macpherson's house at the corner of Bay and Montreal Streets, Kingston, Upper Canada.

1820 Hugh Macdonald opens his first Kingston store.

1822 Five-year-old James Macdonald dies at the hands of a servant.

1822 John A. starts primary school.

1824 Macdonald family moves to Hay Bay, Bay of Quinte. Hugh Macdonald opens a new shop.

1824 Macdonald family moves to Glenora, Prince Edward County, and Hugh Macdonald buys a mill.

1824 John A., age nine, is sent to Midland District Grammar School in Kingston.

1829 John A. attends Rev. Cruickshank's Grammar School.

1829 John A. travels to York (Toronto) to write the exam that will enable him to become an apprentice lawyer.

1830 John A. begins career as an articled lawyer for George Mackenzie.

1830 The first cooking stove is manufactured in Upper Canada by Joseph Van Nostrand.

1831 *The Cook Not Mad, or Rational Cookery* is published in Kingston, Upper Canada (first Canadian cookbook).

1832 Rideau Canal is completed, linking Ottawa with rest of Upper Canada and St. Lawrence Seaway.

1832 John A. moves to Napanee to manage law office.

1833 John A., age eighteen, takes over the law practice of his cousin Lowther Pennington Macpherson.

1833/34 Kingston Penitentiary is under construction. Opens June 1, 1835 as the Provincial Penitentiary of Upper Canada.

1834 Cholera epidemic in Kingston results in about three hundred deaths (approximately ten percent of the population), including George Mackenzie.

1835 John A. opens a law practice at 171 Wellington Street, Kingston.

1835 John A. lives at 110-112 Rideau Street, Kingston.

1836 February 6—John A. (twenty-one years old) passes the bar exam.

1837 Eighteen-year-old Victoria ascends to the throne in Britain.

1837/38 Rebellions of 1837 and 1838 take place.

1838 Unprovoked raids by a group from American territory attack eastern Upper Canada.

1839 John A. becomes a director of Kingston's Commercial Bank.

1841 Kingston becomes the capital of the new province, which unites Canada East (now Quebec) and Canada West (now Ontario).

1841 October 16—Queen's University officially founded.

1842 John A. travels to England and meets cousin Isabella Clark.

1843 John A. elected as Kingston alderman. Serves from 1843 to 1846.

1843 September 1—John A. marries Isabella Clark.

1844 John A. elected to the House of Assembly of Upper Canada to represent Kingston.

1844 Government moves from Kingston to Montreal.

1845 Isabella leaves Kingston for a three-year sojourn in the USA.

1847 John A. appointed to the Cabinet.

1847 August 2—son John Alexander Macdonald is born.

1848 John A. moves his family to Bellevue House, Kingston.

1848 September 21— thirteen-month-old John dies.

1849 John A. moves his law office to 343 King Street East, Kingston.

1850 March 13—second son, Hugh John, is born.

1852 John A. moves his family to Brock Street, Kingston.

1855 Catharine Parr Traill's book, *The Canadian Settlers' Guide* is published in Toronto.

1856 John A. moves to Toronto.

1857 John A. becomes Premier of the Province of Canada and appoints a Cabinet.

1857 December 28—Isabella dies of an unspecified illness.

1858 February—Queen Victoria chooses Ottawa for the seat of Parliament in Canada.

1860 February—John A. invites eight hundred guests to a Valentine's Day gala dinner in the music hall of the St. Louis Hotel in Quebec City.

1860 John A. moves his offices to 93 Clarence Street, Kingston.

1861 *Mrs. Beeton's Book of Household Management* is published in England.

1861 American Civil War begins.

1862 May 20—the Militia Bill is defeated and John A. submits his resignation.

1862 October 24—Helen Shaw Macdonald (John A.'s mother) dies.

1864 The Charlottetown Conference (September 1-9) and Quebec Conference (October 10-27) pave the way for a union of the British North American colonies.

1865 John A. leases Heathfield (now demolished) in Portsmouth Village, his official residence until 1878.

1867 February 18—John A. marries his second wife, Jamaican-born Susan Agnes Bernard.

1867 July 1—The Dominion of Canada is formed and the British North America (BNA) Act is ratified by the Parliaments of Canada and Britain. Four provinces are included: Ontario, Quebec, Nova Scotia, and New Brunswick.

1867 July 1—John A. is designated first prime minister of Canada and is knighted. Agnes becomes Lady Macdonald.

1867 August 20—Conservative Party and Sir John are elected with a majority.

1869 February 8—Daughter Mary is born with the condition hydrocephaly.

1869 The Dominion of Canada purchases the Northwest Territories from the Hudson's Bay Company.

1870 Manitoba becomes fifth province to join Canada.

1871 British Columbia becomes sixth province to join Canada.

1872 October 12—Conservative Party and Sir John elected with a minority.

1873 Sir John plans the North West Mounted Police, which quickly becomes known as the Mounties.

1873 Prince Edward Island (PEI) becomes the seventh province to join Canada.

1873 November 5—Macdonald government defeated in Pacific Scandal.

1873 November 6—Macdonald resigns.

1878 September 17—Conservatives and Sir John elected with a majority on strength of National Policy.

1879 National policy implemented to provide protection for Canada's manufacturing and processing industries.

1879 Thomas Edison invents the incandescent light bulb.

1882 June 20—Conservative Party elected with a majority, but Sir John loses seat in Kingston and is elected instead in Victoria, BC.

1882 May 4—Old Guard gala dinner in honour of Sir John.

1883 Sir John and Lady Agnes move to Earnscliffe in Ottawa.

1884 Grand gala dinner held by the Liberal-Conservative Party in honour of Sir John.

1885 November 7—Last spike of the Canadian Pacific Railway (CPR) driven, in Craigellachie, BC, five years ahead of schedule.

1885 Riel Rebellion results in hanging death of Louis Riel, charged with sedition. Sir John loses popularity.

1886 Sir John and Lady Agnes travel across Canada on CPR.

1887 February 22—Conservative Party and Sir John elected with a fourth majority government.

1891 March 5—Conservatives and Sir John are elected with a fifth majority government.

1891 June 6—Sir John Macdonald dies in Ottawa. Official cause of death is listed as stroke. His body is returned to Kingston to be buried in the Cataraqui Cemetery.

Introduction

We Canadians have been lucky. Things could have been so different. Canada—the true north strong and free, the almighty country stretching from sea to sea to sea—came perilously close to not being a nation at all.

If Hugh Macdonald had been a better businessman, his cotton manufacturing company might have thrived and he wouldn't have sought to leave his native Scotland and take his wife and four children to live in Upper Canada. As it was, Hugh Macdonald had a propensity for talk and a penchant for drinking alcohol but little in the way of business savvy. His cotton business failed. And then his next venture foundered as well. Fearing destitution and drawn by the promise of a new frontier, Hugh Macdonald packed up shop in Glasgow and bought passage for his family to cross the Atlantic Ocean and join their relatives in a place called Kingston, Upper Canada. The year was 1820.

John Alexander Macdonald, born either January 10 or January 11, 1815, was the middle child of five born to Hugh and Helen (Shaw) Macdonald. Just five years old when he left Scotland, the young John A. already showed signs of sharing his father's genial nature, charm, curiosity, and conversational abilities, and his mother's sharp memory and fierce intelligence. One brother had died in infancy, making John the eldest male amongst the four remaining children. The family, including John's older sister, Margaret, and younger siblings, James and Louisa, boarded the steerage compartment of the *Earl of*

Buckinghamshire, bound for Upper Canada, anticipating adventures at sea and a new beginning in an unknown land.

Nobody aboard the ship could ever have imagined the remarkable future that lay ahead of John Alexander Macdonald, who would go on to become the principal founding father and leader of the newborn nation of Canada, and one of the most important people in the history of the country — a country that just might not have happened without him. His staggering list of accomplishments is almost as unparalleled as his addiction to alcohol and his many foibles.

Sir John has been called the man to whom we owe our nationhood, and for this Hugh Macdonald's misfortune became a nation's fortune instead.

Over the years, Macdonald has also been referred to as a rascal and self-deprecating prankster who once planted a dead horse in the pulpit of a local church; a seedy-looking old beggar; a horrendous drunk who was bodily removed from the House of Commons on at least one occasion; an ingenious lawyer and clever, corrupt politician; an artful dodger; a racist; a devoted and caring father, husband and friend; a man's man; and a gracious and flirtatious ladies' man. His own sister once said that he was "the ugliest man in Canada."

Sir John was devoted to each of his two wives yet was said to have a penchant for women in general and particularly for women of "dubious distinction." One of his closest and oldest friends was an uneducated Irish barmaid who rose from rags to riches and is buried next to the Macdonald family plot in the Cataraqui Cemetery in Kingston.

Macdonald is said to have starved the West, sent toxic rations to First Nations People, and to have been a racist. He made some serious and grave errors of judgment, including his mistreatment of migrant workers and his dealings with Louis Riel, the Métis, and First Nations people.

John A. Macdonald was a long way from perfect. He was a product of his times even though, in many ways, he was surprisingly forward thinking.

He lived a life filled with tragedy, and yet he remained buoyant thanks in part to the profound resources of his personality. A voracious reader who read widely, from politics to Trollope to poetry, he was an intellectual but never pretentious, arrogant yet not a snob, remembered people whom he had met only once, and was almost always in possession of an excellent sense of humour. He was devoted to his mother and kept a photograph of her on his desk at all times. He was dedicated to his sisters. He was an early feminist, in favour of equal rights for women and was thought to have coined the term *shero* for female hero. In 1885, he was the first leader in the world to propose that women should be permitted to vote. He was brave and bold. He was a visionary, yet he was also highly pragmatic. He had a rare gift for friendship that knew no limits: neither age, gender, politics, class, nor ethnicity stood in the way of his many deep, lasting, and abiding relationships. Most of all it was said of Sir John that people liked him because he liked people.

Sir John's Table traverses the colourful life of John A. Macdonald from the grim rations he endured on his passage as a young boy from Scotland to Upper Canada, through his boyhood years of stealing fish and scarfing down fairy cakes, to his adult life as a lawyer, husband, father, and politician and the extravagant high teas, campaign picnics, and dinner parties he loved to throw. It was a journey that began with hardtack and suspicious-looking, watered-down stew served in filthy conditions; it culminated in the finest champagne at grand state galas held in his honour.

These are the food stories of Sir John, an intelligent, sociable man, full of bonhomie. Here is a character who loved his family, surrounded himself with lots of company, and adored a party.

This is not a cookbook but a tale of our gastronomic past, found in old recipe books, tales of pioneer life in Canada, and by reading the back stories of Sir John A. Macdonald's life and the context of nineteenth-century society in Upper Canada. Cooking, like history, is by its very nature an act of construction.

Food was a constant challenge for the pioneers and settlers who had much to learn in the wilderness and harsh conditions of life in early Canada. It was especially challenging for the four out of five new immigrants living in rural settings. Ensuring a constant food supply was an all-consuming task for most early settlers. This test of survival played an important role in the economic growth and social development of the colony. Culinary history, a topic once largely overlooked, is increasingly well respected as an aspect of cultural heritage.

Food stories are, after all, our stories—the *real* stories of our lives.

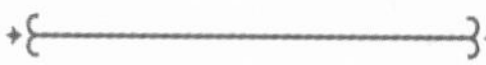

A NOTE ABOUT THE RECIPES

The recipes selected for this book had to meet three criteria: they had to be authentic; feasible, in that the ingredients are actually obtainable; and edible. For example, recipes for collared calf's head, calf's head turtle fashion, calves head hash, pig's head souse, as well as cow heels and pig's ears, scalloped frogs, and pearl ash (pot ash) cake are not included here on the grounds that even if the ingredients were to be sourced, the results would likely be considered inedible.

Most of the recipes included are taken from old books and attributed accordingly. They are used here verbatim, without changes or explanations. Often directions are incomplete, lacking oven temperatures and cooking times. This is because during the early to mid-1800s, most Canadian families used a fire to do their cooking. Oven temperatures were not relevant. Likewise the measurements and instructions given in the recipes have not been modified or metricated. Modern variations of most of the recipes included here can easily be found. But for those who are interested in Canadian culinary history, they can rest assured that these recipes (or "receipts," as they were then known) are authentic and exactly what Helen Shaw Macdonald would have used to feed her family.

A NOTE ABOUT TERMINOLOGY

Upper and Lower Canada / Canada East and Canada West

The Constitutional Act of 1791 created the areas of Upper and Lower Canada, today's Ontario and Quebec respectively. In 1841, the two Canadas were joined to form the Province of Canada, whereupon Upper Canada became Canada West and Lower Canada became Canada East. The terms were used interchangeably throughout the period prior to Confederation.

Canadian Currency: Pounds versus Dollars

Each region of what is now known as Canada had its own system of government, currency, and postage stamps. In 1841, the new Province of Canada adopted the Canadian pound. One pound (£1) was worth 16 shillings and 5.3 pence. In 1858, the Province of Canada converted to a decimal system and brought in the Canadian dollar, the same system of currency still in use today.

CHAPTER ONE

Passage to Upper Canada: Bring Your Own Biscuits

1815–20

John A. Macdonald was just four years old when he made his first "public" speech. While his parents were hosting visitors in the sitting room, the children were sent to the kitchen to occupy themselves, out of sight of the adults. John A. promptly climbed atop the kitchen table and began a performance for his captive audience of siblings and friends. In between his words and wild gesticulations with both his arms and his legs, he managed to propel himself off the table, landing on a chair and gashing his forehead badly enough that the resulting scar was still visible upon his death. Perhaps his early precociousness was the reason his mother, Helen Shaw Macdonald, was so fond of saying, "Mark my words, John will make more than the ordinary man."[1]

In June 1820, a year after John A.'s maiden speech, and two years after the 49th parallel had been named the border between British North America and the United States, Hugh and Helen Macdonald gathered their belongings and their four children, Margaret, John A., James, and Louisa, along with an orphaned cousin, Maria, and Hugh Macdonald's elderly, frail mother and set sail for the New World. They were leaving Scotland aboard the *Earl of Buckinghamshire,* destined for the port of Quebec, and finally, their new home in Kingston, Upper Canada.

The Macdonalds travelled below deck, in steerage class, alongside the majority of the ship's other 350 passengers. For forty-two days, the eight Macdonald family members endured no privacy except that provided by a lice-riddled blanket that they suspended around the 1.5-metre square area, stacked with bunk beds, that constituted their home during the Atlantic crossing. The only toilets on the ship were two privies. There was a dearth of food. The poorly ventilated steerage compartment was sour with the pungent smell of unwashed bodies, damp dirty clothes, a general lack of sanitation, sewage, sweat and vomit, and rotting food. Many of the passengers were desperately seasick. Others had dysentery and respiratory infections. There was no source of light or fresh air other than what filtered in through cracks. The only water for washing was sea water. Rats were rampant. Everything was damp and dirty, and at times the passengers sloshed through filthy water underfoot.

These early, over-crowded vessels were known as "coffin ships" because so many people died onboard. It was not until 1847 that modest sanitation regulations were put in place to increase the likelihood of safe passage on ocean-going vessels. Even so, steerage passengers were lucky if there was one privy to every one hundred passengers and adequate fresh water for drinking.

Food in steerage consisted primarily of watered-down oatmeal and molasses, hardtack, and dubious, unsavoury stews, often made with horse meat or the leftovers from the first- and second-class dining rooms. There was no dining room for the steerage class. Passengers lined up for their food, doled from huge kettles into their dinner pails. The bread was often mouldy and virtually inedible. It was not an unknown practice for captains to deliberately feed the steerage passengers food that would make them ill so that they would not demand their full rations. But Helen Macdonald, who was kind, capable, and resourceful, had the foresight to bring food supplies for her family, including bread (likely bannock), cheese, and biscuits. In this way, she was able to keep them somewhat healthy and provide at least a small measure of comfort during the six-week crossing.

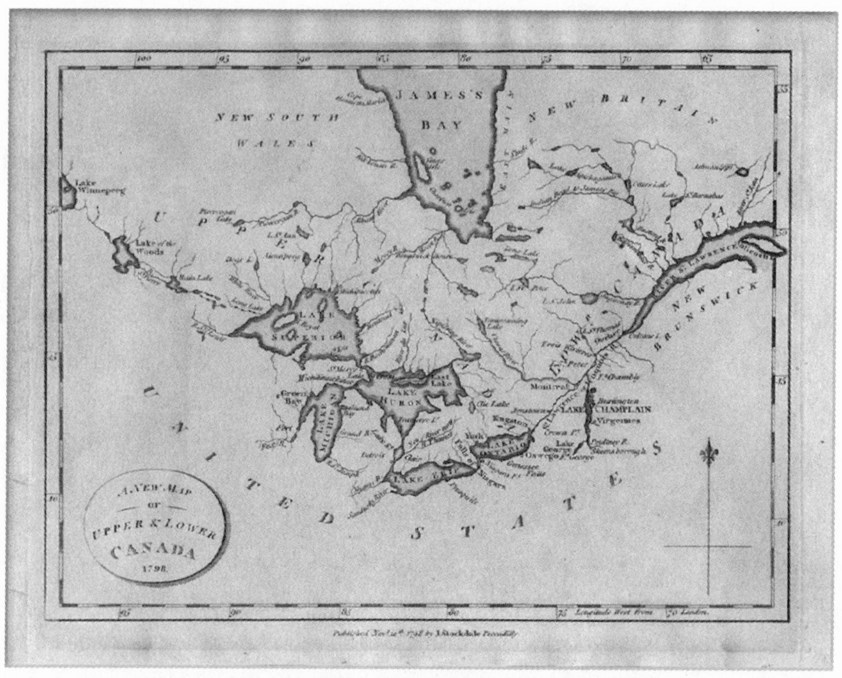

Map of Upper and Lower Canada, 1798

By all accounts, John A. was a lively, happy child, fond of playing with his siblings, and when left to his own devices, he entertained himself with the solitary card game patience. Amongst the squalor of steerage class, it isn't likely that he and his siblings would have had much opportunity for any kind of play. Their main enjoyment would have come from their brief periods above deck, where they were allowed to walk around in specific areas but not to mix with the first- and second-class passengers.

After forty-two harsh days at sea, the *Earl of Buckinghamshire* arrived in Quebec City, and its weary passengers disembarked. The second part of the Macdonalds' journey was almost as hard as the first. They travelled up the St. Lawrence River aboard *bateaux* and Durham boats, which were open to the elements and sometimes under sail but more often poled, pushed, or pulled, and sometimes dragged by both men and oxen. At night, they hauled the boats ashore and slept alongside the river. They lacked any kind of adequate sanitation or shelter; they cooked their meals on open fires and slept as best they could amidst the mosquitos and wildlife—though they were likely too tired to care.

There are varying accounts of the duration of this second stage of the journey to Kingston, but one thing is certain: the Macdonald family were in transit for at least nine weeks from the day they left Scotland, a journey that would now take closer to nine hours and still elicit serious grumbling.

On August 13, 1820, the Macdonalds arrived at the two-storey home of Helen Macdonald's stepsister, Anna Shaw, her husband, Colonel Donald Macpherson, and their eight children. Here, at the corner of Bay and Montreal streets in Kingston, Upper Canada, the travel weary Macdonalds were finally able to bathe, wash their clothes, rest, and enjoy some wholesome food before establishing themselves in their own quarters. They spent three months living in the Macpherson home before finding a suitable location for their new general store.

In this period, Kingston was rough and rude and had a reputation for debauchery. It was a town rife with drunkards and prostitutes. It was also one of the most important settlements in Upper Canada because of its strategic location at the intersection of the St. Lawrence River and the Great Lakes. It was larger than York, which later became Toronto. With a population of about 3,500, Kingston was home to Fort Henry, a naval shipyard, some handsome and substantial homes, some good schools, shops, St. Andrew's Presbyterian Church, a newspaper, and at least seventy-eight taverns.

Even the wealthiest homes in Upper and Lower Canada in the early 1800s were primitive. This was an age before indoor plumbing, public waterworks, sewers, and electricity. It was an era of candles, oil and kerosene lamps, chamber pots, outdoor privies, wood and coal fires, and in urban areas, carters who delivered water. It wasn't until the mid-1800s that cities in Upper and Lower Canada began building municipal waterworks for the supply of safe water. Electricity and lighting came later still.

THE IMMIGRANT KITCHEN AND DIET

Like much of Upper Canada, Kingston was populated by English and Scottish immigrants. They favoured the cuisine they already knew, which was a diet heavy on starch and stodge, as well as meat, fish, game, and well-cooked vegetables. In addition they enjoyed oatmeal, plenty of potatoes, bread, bannock, butter, cheese, and baked desserts, including steamed puddings, pastries, and of course, shortbread.

Food was a challenge for all, although those in town fared better than the settlers on the land where provisions were hard to come by and conditions were harsh. Preoccupation with sustenance was a necessity for survival and much of the population was involved in some way with the production and procurement of food. Eighty percent of settlers were farmers or independent fisherman—an industrious group who built their own houses, grew almost all their own food, and made nearly everything in their possession from vinegar, wine, and yeast to furniture, clothes, brooms, quilts, soap, and candles.

The Macdonalds were doubly fortunate in that, being shopkeepers, they had access to a wider variety of groceries and supplies than many of their neighbours. As well, the Macpherson relatives were well off and well connected in Kingston. With their new business and the right patrons, Helen Macdonald would have been able to continue to feed her family as well or better than she ever had.

A surprising list of commodities was available for those in town who could afford such luxuries. Readily available were flour, cornmeal, oatmeal, rice, pearl barley, sugar, gelatin powder, raisins, currants, citron, capers, salt, pepper, tea, coffee, olive oil, anchovy paste, lard, suet, butter, vinegar, beer, wine, maple syrup, molasses, and biscuits. Various spices including curry powder, cayenne pepper, cloves, parsley, sage, cinnamon, mace, mustard powder, and ginger were all in common usage. Casks of salt pork, salted beef, and bacon were regular provisions. Fish, meat, eggs, butter, and fresh fruit and vegetables were available according to the season. Though not common, lemons and oranges were highly prized and obtainable when ships arrived from overseas. Cocoa powder, primarily used for drinking chocolate, was developed in the early 1800s; solid chocolate for eating was not widely available until the late 1800s. Flour, which was sometimes in scarce supply, been one commodity that the Macdonalds had in plenty. This enabled the family to eat good breads, pastry, puddings, and biscuits.

Bannock, a traditional Scottish quick bread, was a mainstay of the diet of early explorers, fur traders, voyageurs, and settlers of North America. It was prized for its portability and durability—a perfect food for travelling. While it was widely believed that the Scottish introduced bannock to the indigenous people of North America, plenty of evidence exists that that this was not so and that grain was available to the aboriginal tribes for a similar style of bread. References to bannock also appear in the early journals of the Hudson's Bay Company, which set up posts in northern Canada in the seventeenth century.

Early bannocks were small, heavy, flat, dry cakes made with oatmeal, barley, or cornmeal along with water and then cooked on a griddle over a fire with whatever grease or fat was available. Prior to the 1800s, bannock was unleavened, unlike bread, which was leavened with yeast. The only other early leavening agent in common use in North America was pearl ash, a purified version of potash made from lye. Pearl ash was replaced by sodium bicarbonate, or baking soda, by the 1840s. Baking powder, which is a mixture of sodium bicarbonate and tartaric acid, was introduced shortly after and subsequent recipes for bannock are leavened, making bannock more like a contemporary scone.

In the 1800s, homes in Upper and Lower Canada had a fireplace for heating and cooking, and some had a small oven that was a hole in the wall with a door that was heated by the fireplace stones. Settlers baked bannock either on a griddle suspended over the fire, or in the bake oven, in a cast-iron pan. From 1830 on, as wood-fired cast iron stoves became available in Upper Canada, cooking and baking processes were slowly transformed.

The first cookbook produced in Canada was *The Cook Not Mad, or Rational Cookery: Being a Collection of Original and Selected Receipts,* published in Kingston in 1831 by James Macfarlane. It was essentially an American cookbook that was given a Canadian cover. Cooking temperatures, accurate measures, and cooking times were left almost entirely to the imagination.

Like most early cookbooks, *The Cook Not Mad* made no reference to bannock because it was a basic recipe that everyone knew. Early cookbooks were considered a luxury item and often contained a diverse collection of recipes, household hints and advice, and tips for caring for the sick. Catharine Parr Traill, the English emigrant who wrote about her life as a settler in Canada, mentions bannock only once in all her writing and even this is with a disparaging remark: "Careful people, of course, who know this peculiarity, are on the watch, being aware of the ill consequences of heavy bread, or having no bread but bannocks in the house."[2]

Nonetheless, bannock was essential for survival and has a long and important history in both Scottish and First Nations cultures. Undoubtedly Helen Macdonald would have brought bannock with her aboard the *Earl of Buckinghamshire*, as well as shortbread, another standby of the Scottish kitchen. The Scottish appetite for shortbread is well known, and while there are variations of shortbread in other cuisines, it was the Scottish who developed the biscuit to an art form. Shortbread dates back to the twelfth century and was said to have been a favourite of Mary, Queen of Scots (1542-87). Walkers Shortbread remains Scotland's largest exporter of food, shipping its biscuits all the way around the globe.

Early recipes for shortbread use a formula of three-parts flour, two-parts butter, and one-part sugar. This traditional shortbread is adapted from the old Scottish recipe used today by Sir John's Public House, in Kingston, Ontario. The pub occupies the original premises of Macdonald's law practice, where he made his living from 1849 to 1860. In many countries, the homes and business sites of first leaders are made into museums and national historic landmarks. Perhaps it's fitting that the business office of Canada's Scottish-born first leader, Sir John, a legendary drinker, is now a pub.

SIR JOHN'S SHORTBREAD

2 ½ cups (250 grams) unbleached all-purpose flour
¾ cup (145 grams) sugar
1 cup (225 grams) salted butter, well chilled

Preheat oven to 325°F (165°C).

Combine sugar and flour in large bowl. Grate the well-chilled butter and stir into the flour and sugar until the mixture is fine and crumbly. Press into an 8-by-8-inch square glass pan. Prick the surface with a fork.

Bake for 20–25 minutes or until pale golden — not brown. Cool and cut into fingers.

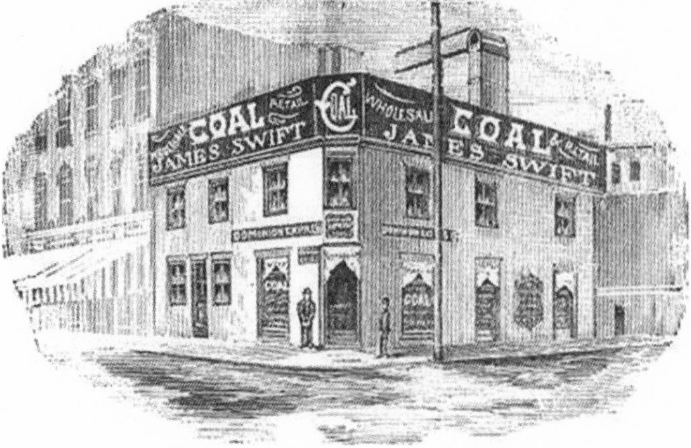

Hugh Macdonald's store in Kingston

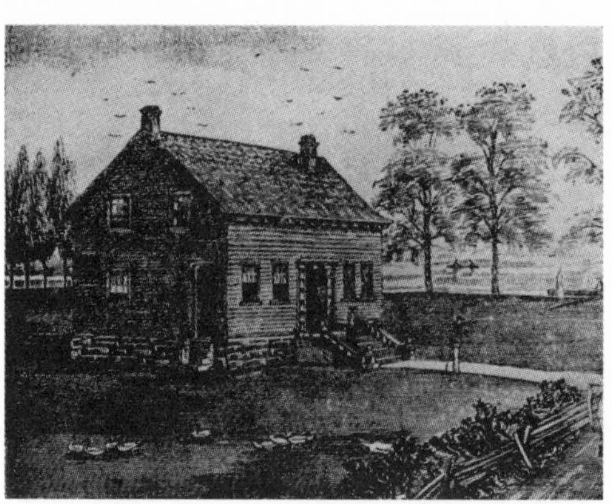

The Macdonald homestead at Adolphustown

CHAPTER TWO

Boyhood: A Fish Tale

1820–25

Three months after their arrival in Upper Canada, Hugh Macdonald set up a general store on King Street in Kingston, where he sold an eclectic collection of groceries, liquor, gun paraphernalia, and assorted hardware. An advertisement in the *Kingston Chronicle* on July 3, 1821, informed readers of new "fancy goods suitable for the season," and went on to list commonly available stock, including "Wines, Jamaica Spirits, Brandy, Gin, Shrub and Vinegar, Powder and Shot, English Window Glass and Putty."

Initially, the family lived above the shop and enjoyed adequate provisions from their own store. For a while, at least, their new life in Upper Canada was off to a good start.

Unfortunately, the shop failed rather quickly. Undaunted by another business fiasco, Hugh set up a new shop on Store Street (now known as Princess Street). In short order, this shop also began to flounder.

It was during this time that John A. witnessed the violent death of his younger brother James, who at five years old was brutally beaten by a drunken servant named Kennedy. The Macdonald family kept the story of James's death a secret, and it was never talked about until many decades later when Sir John finally broke the silence. Amongst the varying accounts of what transpired, one story seems consistent. James had apparently tried to accompany his parents on an evening walk but was sent home to remain with the other children. What happened next is less clear, but it seems that the children's caregiver, Kennedy, a secret drinker, reacted to the crying boy by either shoving him into the iron grate of a fireplace or beating him, or perhaps both. In any case, shortly after this incident James died of internal injuries. Incredibly, the family did not press charges and merely ran a short, sad obituary in the Kingston paper acknowledging the boy's death.

Following James's horrifying death and the failures of Hugh Macdonald's Kingston ventures, the family decided to relocate to Hay Bay, on the Bay of Quinte, west of Kingston. By 1824, Hugh opened a shop in Hay Bay and was the local agent for the *Kingston Chronicle*. The family settled into their home on the banks of Lake Ontario, and the three children walked together on the daily six-mile round trip between home and school.

During the Hay Bay era, the young John A. was out one summer day, exploring the local waterfront when he ran into a man fishing from the shore. Nine-year-old John walked up, thrust out his hand, and introduced himself to the fisherman, admiring his catch and telling the man his life story. They talked for a while until the fisherman cast his line again. Just as soon as the man had turned his back on the boy and returned his attention to his work, John A. grabbed the biggest of his fish—a large black bass—and ran for home. The fisherman shouted out after him to no avail.

Years later, in 1837, when John A. was speaking at a political gathering in the Adolphustown Town Hall, Mr. Guy Casey was waiting for his opportunity. When his moment came, he rose and told the story of a young boy named John A. Macdonald who once stole his fish and ran for home. Mr. Casey then demanded that John A. publicly acknowledge his crime. The crowd turned expectantly to John A., who bowed his head solemnly and said,

> Mr. Chairman and yeoman of Adolphustown, what my old neighbour has told you about the theft of his beautiful fish is absolutely true. I can recall as though it were but yesterday

> how frightened I was at that unearthly yell of our good friend, which almost caused me to drop the fish so as to make better speed, but I managed to hold onto it when I saw he was not chasing me. I was clean out of breath when I burst into the house and fell headlong with it on the floor, and gasped for breath as I told my father where I found it, and that there were lots more like it where this came from. I humbly beg your pardon, Guy, and my only regret is that I can't steal another one like it here tonight and have it for breakfast in the morning. Mother said it was the best black bass she ever cooked.[3]

Not surprisingly, John A.'s flattery, honesty, and charm appeased Guy Casey and won over the crowd. This great fish tale, one of John A.'s early public speeches, brought the house down.

THE IMPORTANCE OF FISH AND GAME

Any inexpensive source of food was sought after, and fish and game were no exception. The early settlers initially learned to hunt and fish from the First Nations. For thousands of years, the aboriginal people had fished using spears, nets, hooks, traps and longlines and hunted with snare traps, spears, and later, with bows and arrows. They treated the animals and fish with respect and took only what they needed. Almost nothing went to waste.

The abundance of fish and game was a boon to new settlers whose principal protein source would otherwise have been salted pork — a dish that quickly grew monotonous to the palate. They began to hunt deer, moose, rabbit, hare, goose, duck, wild pigeon, wild turkey, quail, ptarmigan, partridge, and bear. Raccoon, beaver, porcupine, and even black squirrel were also sought after. As the settlers moved further west to the prairies, they depended on venison, elk, moose, bighorn sheep, lynx, rabbit, gopher, prairie hen, goose, and most importantly of all, buffalo, until the extermination of the herds, beginning in 1875. The settlers brought with them guns and ammunition, and what they didn't hunt for themselves, they traded with the First Nations, offering in exchange flour and salted pork.

Fishing was equally important. Beginning when the first Europeans reached the east coast of North America and found the waters teeming with fish, shellfish, and seals, a new industry was born. There are stories of fish being so plentiful that one only needed to dip a net in the water in order to have food for dinner. It was not unusual for families to lay up six or eight barrels of fish to last through the winter, although ice fishing was common for those in close enough proximity to a frozen lake. Fishing was not just an industry but also a practical and productive pastime. Cod, halibut, haddock, mackerel, pollock, sardines, herring, lobsters, mussels, and oysters came from the sea coasts. Inland, the lakes and rivers supplied pike, pickerel, muskellunge, eels, whitefish, largemouth bass, mullet, lake herring, sturgeon, burbot, carp, shad, and wall-eye. Smaller fish like salmon, trout, perch, sunfish, and small mouth bass were also prevalent. Whitefish, which were abundant in Upper Canada lakes, were a universal favourite, prized for their rich, fine flavour.

The Black bass that John A. stole from Guy Casey was likely a largemouth bass, reported to grow to up to a metre (or just over three feet) in length, though it would be rare to find one of that size now.

This recipe for a baked and stuffed black bass is from *The Canadian Home Cookbook*, 1877. It doesn't specify the weight of fish required, but given the amount of stuffing produced with "eight good sized onions," a very large fish is needed. Alternately, cut the amount of stuffing in half. Whole salmon also works well as a substitute for the bass.

BAKED BLACK BASS

Eight good sized onions chopped fine
half that quantity of bread crumbs
butter size of hen's egg
plenty of pepper and salt
mix thoroughly with anchovy sauce until quite red.

Stuff your fish with this compound and pour the rest over it, previously sprinkling with a little red pepper. Shad, pickerel and trout are good the same way.

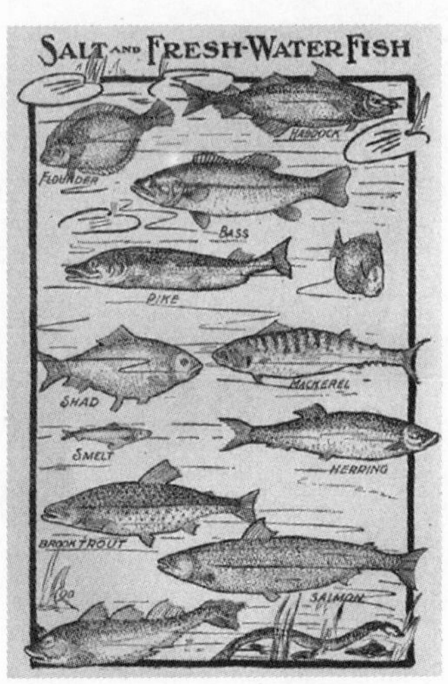

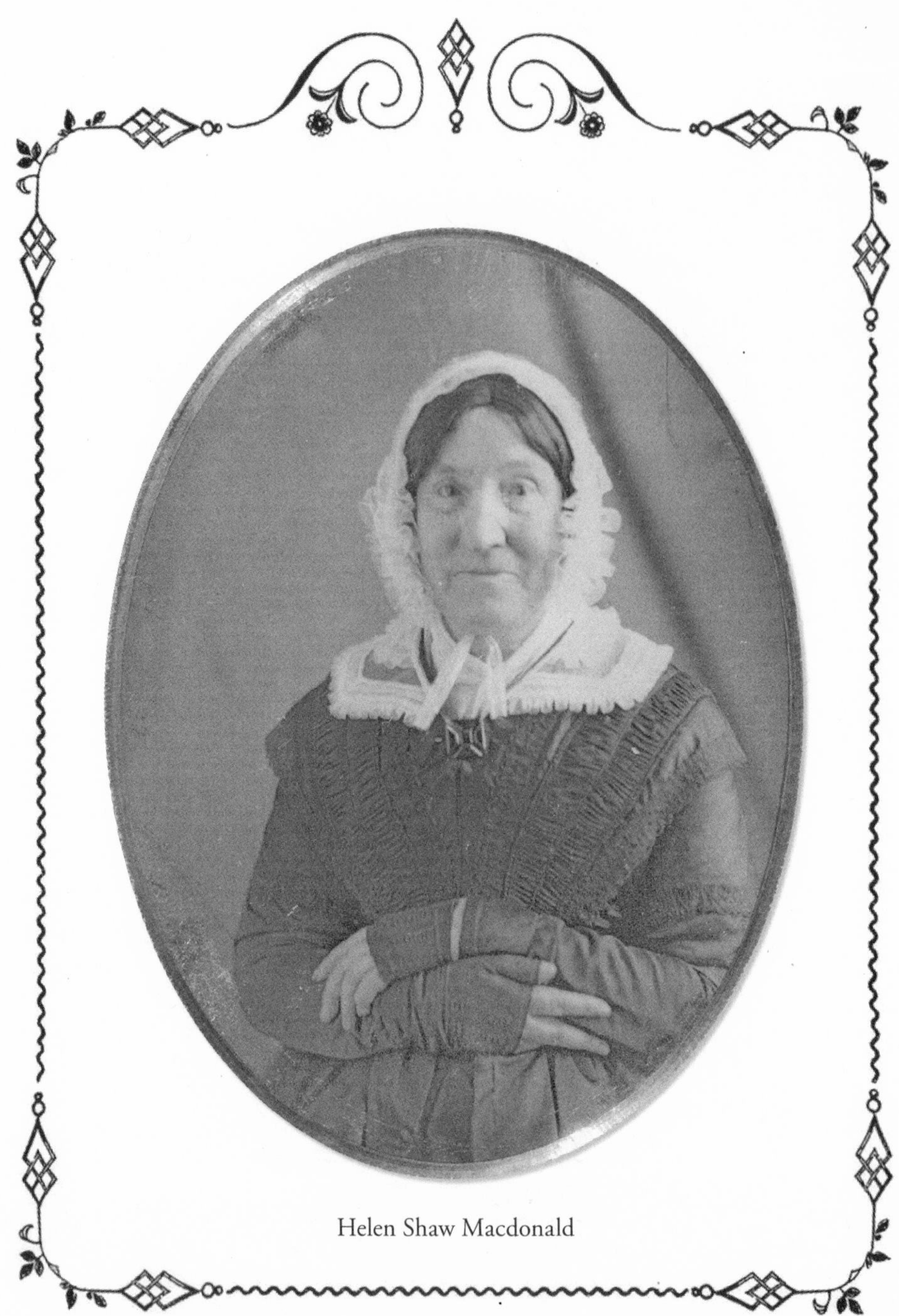
Helen Shaw Macdonald

CHAPTER THREE

School Years: Scarfing Down Puddings

1825–29

"I had no boyhood," John A. Macdonald once said, looking back on his early years. "From the age of fifteen, I began to earn my own living."[4] It was an uncharacteristic lament, for although John A. was subject to occasional despair, he was usually high-spirited and frequently turned his sharp sense of humour upon himself.

In fact, it is true that his boyhood was marred by witnessing the murder of his younger brother, as well as by his father's drinking and business failures, which brought intermittent poverty to the family and frequent moves. At a young age he was sent to Kingston to attend school, which was not so uncommon. Few in the new colonies had an easy life, and many had it as bad or worse. Many young men had to grow up in a hurry and help support their families. Only a very few, from the wealthiest families, attended university, and often they were sent to Britain.

John A. had one advantage throughout most of his life that helped override everything else: he had the unconditional love and support of his mother — a fact that almost every one of his many biographers has commented upon. Helen Shaw Macdonald was solid in every sense of the word. A stout, practical woman, she was devoted to her family. Helen Macdonald was selfless and intelligent with an excellent memory and a droll sense of humour. She was also lively and spontaneous and possessed of a great sense of fun. Once, upon hearing bagpipes coming down the road, Helen ran out of the house and danced a jig in the street. Throughout her life, her children remained devoted to her, and many episodes of John A.'s life can be put together from his ongoing correspondence with his mother. Later in his life, John A. always kept a photograph of her close at hand.

In 1824, the family moved again, this time to Glenora in Prince Edward County, where Hugh bought a mill. For a time the family enjoyed some financial stability while the mill provided at least enough income for Hugh and Helen Macdonald to begin to save a bit of money.

Despite lamenting about his boyhood years, John was by all accounts a good-natured boy, always quick with a joke or a pun or a practical joke. He took pleasure in reading, enjoyed company, and loved his sisters. He was not immune, though, to enjoying a bit of teenaged trouble-making. As one of his friends said of him, "There wasn't much fun that John A. wasn't up to."[5] Once, upon heading home from some late night activities in Kingston, Macdonald and his friends noticed the roadway was covered in limestone pieces in preparation for making a street. It was one o'clock in the morning—late enough that the city was cloaked in darkness and still early enough that the group of lads had energy to spare.

Macdonald immediately took charge: he figured that the stone could be used to create a decent sized wall. Scanning the immediate area, he pointed out grocer Jemmy Williamson's doorway.

"It would not look amiss with a nice new stone front added to it," he said.[6]

For two hours, in near complete silence, the boys removed every stone from the roadway and built a wall, seven feet long and eight feet high, entirely blocking Jemmy Williamson's front door. Then, before they headed home, the boys threw stones at the upstairs windows. Williamson eventually woke up, came downstairs, and threw open his door only to be confronted by the wall of stone. He was heard crying out, "My God! What sin have I committed that this horror should fall upon me?"—at which point John A. and his chums scampered off to find their beds.

Macdonald passed the store the next day and found the wall gone. Later on in his life, he recalled the incident, saying that if he hadn't read about it in the newspaper, he would have thought the whole thing a dream.[7]

One night, John A. and his friends were out walking through the village of Picton when, to their great delight, they found a dead horse. They propped the horse up in the pulpit of the local Methodist Church and waited for the elderly sexton to enter the church to light the lamps. When the unsuspecting sexton saw the animal, hooves upon the pulpit, he ran screaming from the building, claiming that he'd seen the devil himself. The local constable was brought in and promptly called up the usual suspects, including the young John A. Macdonald.

Another time John A. and his friends erected a fence across the Main Street of Picton in order to stop a horse and driver who routinely galloped through town. They were performing a public service, they thought. The horse was maimed, and a suspect who had nothing to do with the case was on the verge of conviction when John A.'s conscience got the better of him, and he came forward and confessed. Somehow he managed to get away with a mere reprimand. It was said that, in later years, this episode served John A. as a reminder of the dangers of circumstantial evidence.

The pranks, however, were not restricted to late-night practical jokes with his mates. Once, his sisters, Louisa and Margaret, and a friend of theirs were about to head off for an afternoon row on Lake Ontario when John A. noticed they had climbed aboard the boat without the oars. He grabbed the opportunity to shove the boat off the shore, casting them adrift in the lake. The girls yelled and shouted until their mother came to see what the fuss was about. Luckily for John A., the wind brought the girls back to shore without incident.

On another occasion, John A. and his sisters were playing soldiers—as they often did—with John A. playing captain and assigning various duties to the girls. Louisa refused to play along, which caused John A. to grab a gun from the wall and point it at her head, threatening to shoot her if she did not comply. It was Margaret who intervened and took the gun away. Only later was it discovered by their father that the gun was loaded.

Despite his antics, or perhaps because of them, Hugh and Helen Macdonald decided to spend a good portion of their savings to send John A. to Kingston to attend the Midland District Grammar School, where the headmaster, Reverend John Wilson, was a fellow of the University of Oxford. Helen viewed John's education as an investment in the family's future, for she never once doubted that he had great potential. So the Macdonalds paid the seventy pounds annual tuition, and John boarded with his friend, Charles Stuart, in the house of two elderly ladies at 110 Rideau Street, in Kingston.

During his school years in Kingston, the young John A. was a regular visitor at the Macphersons' house, where the Macdonald family had stayed on their arrival in Kingston. John was said to have been drawn by his uncle's library and by the pudding saved for him by Macphersons' youngest daughter, who was said to be delighted with her cousin's capacity for scarfing down slices of pudding and fairy cakes.[8]

A PENCHANT FOR PUDDINGS

Baked, boiled, or steamed puddings were immensely popular in the nineteenth century, and few dinners were complete without one. There were the classics, such as jam roly poly, bread pudding, plum pudding, and rice pudding, and there were staples, such as ginger, apple, and Indian pudding, which was made of cornmeal.

Baked or steamed puddings were generally heavy, starchy desserts, often containing suet or butter, and flour, rice, or cornmeal. They were useful for filling hungry families and were a practical way to stretch out small amounts of expensive ingredients, such as sugar, eggs, spices, and butter, and fresh, dried, or preserved fruit.

Bread pudding was made from leftover stale bread. The dessert is known in almost every culture around the world in some guise, and the first known British version appeared in the literature in John Nott's *Cook's and Confectioner's Dictionary* of 1723. Almost all early North American cookbooks had at least one recipe for bread pudding and some had several, often varied by calling for dried fruit, including currants, raisins, and citron. The version below is from *The Cook Not Mad*, 1831.

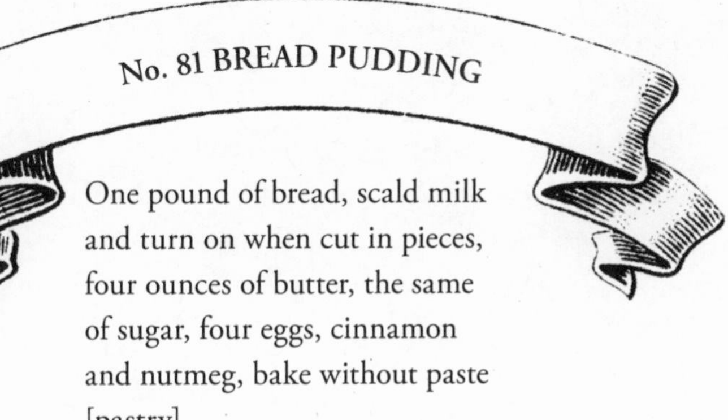

No. 81 BREAD PUDDING

One pound of bread, scald milk and turn on when cut in pieces, four ounces of butter, the same of sugar, four eggs, cinnamon and nutmeg, bake without paste [pastry].

CHAPTER FOUR

Law and Order

1829–32

In 1829, Helen and Hugh Macdonald decided to enrol fourteen-year-old John A. in Reverend John Cruickshank's new, upmarket, coeducational Kingston Grammar School. Cruickshank, a devout Presbyterian, had a reputation not just for cultivating scholastic excellence but also for fostering social ambitions.

Unfortunately, no sooner had John A. settled into his new school than his father's mill business began what now seems like an inevitable descent towards failure. It became apparent that John A.'s school days were limited, even though his father was determined to hang onto the mill for a bit longer, in case his luck changed. Fortunately, through a series of connections, Hugh Macdonald was appointed magistrate for the Midland district, a position that helped him ease his way out of his entrepreneurial endeavours while saving face and earning at least a small income.

John A.'s parents scraped together the funds to send him to Toronto to write the exam that would enable him to begin an apprenticeship as a lawyer. The exam tested his ability in Latin and mathematics. John A. passed without difficulty and returned home to Kingston to finish his final school year. He was popular with the other students, in good measure because of his wit, his ability to tell stories, and his great sense of fun. He was shockingly self-confident, and showed little fear of the masters, holding his own in their society at a time when that was certainly not the norm. He was sociable and intelligent and he was an insatiable reader who remembered everything he ever read. He also liked physical activities, including running, skating, and even dancing. He was a source of great entertainment at school dances; once, upon having forgotten a promised dance to a girl, he threw himself upon the floor, begged her forgiveness, and proclaimed with giddy adolescent immaturity, "Remember, oh remember, the fascination of the turkey."[9] Amongst the laughter, the apology was accepted.

Despite his somewhat unusual appearance, John A. was still sought after by the girls. He was tall, standing at almost six feet (1.8 metres), and he had a narrow, expressive face, a large bulbous nose, deep blue eyes, and coarse, wiry, dark hair. He was charming and respectful with women and girls, which could be attributed to the influence of his mother.

The idea that he should become a lawyer had been planted while he was at Midland Grammar School. Frustrated by the juxtaposition of John A.'s scholastic ability and his lack of discipline and increasingly convoluted and inventive excuses for chronic lateness, a teacher told him that he would make a better lawyer than a clergyman. If the remark was meant to be disparaging, it certainly wasn't taken that way. The idea made sense. The colony was growing, and lawyers were in great demand. Start-up costs were minimal. There was, as yet, no formal educational training required. Articled lawyers were paid a reasonable salary to learn the profession on the job. Hugh Macdonald might not have been a particularly astute businessman but one thing he excelled at was recognizing opportunity, and he agreed that having his son become a lawyer was a brilliant opportunity if ever there was one.

Thus, in 1830, at age fifteen, John A. landed a position as an apprentice to George Mackenzie, one of the most prominent, ambitious, and successful lawyers in the City of Kingston. The Scottish connection was important. Belonging to a clan is a Scottish tradition, and once in the colonies, the Scots became a proud new clan, leaving behind some of their old rivalries and banding together, at least for the most part. As a group, they were hardy, progressive, forward-thinking, fuelled by alcohol, and hell-bent on success.

During the 1800s and early 1900s, the Scots were, collectively, a powerhouse in British North America and elsewhere around the world.

John A.'s Scottish birthright may have given him some benefits, but he was, in fact, a young Upper Canadian lad. He had a tempered, mostly local accent. Fellow Scot Alexander Campbell, who ended up articling under John A. Macdonald before going on to become premier of Ontario, once said of John A. that he was "in tone of voice and manner as thoroughly a Bay of Quinte boy as if he had been born there."[10]

By day, John A. learned the ropes of working in a law office, running various errands and acting as a messenger boy, clerk, and stenographer. By night, he studied the law under the direction of his employer. As was somewhat customary, he boarded with his employer, George Mackenzie, and his wife, Sarah. The Mackenzies lived in a comfortable two-storey stone house on Barrack Street in Kingston. When he could, John A. escaped to the taverns of Kingston. There was no legal drinking age and no real liquor laws to speak of. For the young John A. there were also no limits, that is until one morning when he failed to rouse himself, and Sarah Mackenzie went into his room. Unable to wake him, she drew the blinds completely shut until there was not a glimmer of light in his room. He finally awoke just as the sun was going down again, having missed an entire day of work. Understandably, his employer was not impressed.

When he wasn't in the tavern or the law office or studying, John A. was learning from George and Sarah Mackenzie how a relatively wealthy household might run. The Mackenzies had no children, so they were able to invest a lot of attention in John A. During evenings spent in the Mackenzies' formal dining room, enjoying lavish meals with other prominent Scots, the young man acquired a taste for fine living. Dinner parties and afternoon teas were considered a symbol of gentility. Because the upper class was not doing hard physical labour, unlike most settlers, they tended to eat their dinner, the largest meal of the day, in the evening. Typically dinner was served over several courses, and when company was invited, it could be as many as twelve. Either way, every formal meal began with a savoury soup.

THE SOUP COURSE

Soup was useful to settlers because it was a safe way of using up leftovers at a time when leftover food could not simply be consigned to the refrigerator for storage. In the warmer months the only means of refrigeration came from access to a cool spring or a box buried in the ground. A soup or stock pot provided a method of preserving food safely. Fish and animal bones and vegetable scraps and peelings were boiled down to produce stock which provided vital nutrients, reduced waste, and made a base for soups, stew, and gravy. It was not uncommon for a cook to have a pot of stock simmering over the fire or on the stove continuously for a few days. Kept at a high enough temperature, a soup pot was a safe method for keeping harmful bacteria at bay.

An elegant soup was considered an epicurean necessity. Oyster soup was typically served on special occasions, such as Christmas, New Year's Eve, and gala dinners. Cock-a-leekie (leek, chicken stock, and prunes) and Scotch broth (lamb, vegetables, and barley) were traditional Scottish fare. Early North American cookbooks demonstrate a reverence for "modern recipes" using local and seasonally available ingredients, including pumpkins, potatoes, corn, peas, and parsnips. These root vegetables stored well and were often the main ingredients in soup in winter and spring.

Parsnip soup was popular enough to crop up in various forms in several early cookbooks and later was made even more widely popular with *Mrs. Beeton's Book of Household Management*, first released in 1861. Here is *Mrs. Beeton's* recipe as it first appeared along with the recipe for stock No. 106, called for in the ingredients.

PARSNIP SOUP

141. INGREDIENTS.—1 lb. of sliced parsnips, 2 oz. of butter, salt and cayenne to taste, 1 quart of stock No. 106

Mode.—Put the parsnips into the stewpan with the butter, which has been previously melted, and simmer them till quite tender. Then add nearly a pint of stock, and boil together for half an hour. Pass all through a fine strainer, and put to it the remainder of the stock. Season, boil, and serve immediately.

Time.—2 hours. Average cost, 6d. per quart.
Seasonable from October to April.
Sufficient for 4 persons.

ECONOMICAL STOCK

106. INGREDIENTS.—The liquor in which a joint of meat has been boiled, say 4 quarts; trimmings of fresh meat or poultry, shank-bones, &c., roast-beef bones, any pieces the larder may furnish; vegetables, spices, and the same seasoning as in the foregoing recipe.

Mode.—Let all the ingredients simmer gently for 6 hours, taking care to skim carefully at first. Strain it off, and put by for use.

Time.—6 hours. Average cost, 3d. per quart.

CHAPTER FIVE

Head of the House: A Fortunate Young Man

1832–37

Though no one other than his mother might have predicted it at the time, John A. Macdonald's career was about to begin a speedy ascent on a trajectory that continued for most of his life. Much of John A.'s good fortune and success in the law and in politics could be attributed to his intelligence and good humour. The truth is that there were many factors at play, including his remarkably supportive mother, his Scottish background and the sense of belonging that came with that, and a bit of plain old-fashioned luck.

In fact, at times, other people's misfortunes contributed to John A.'s great fortune. In 1832, George Mackenzie opened a second legal office in Napanee, a town about twenty-five miles west of Kingston, and he installed John A. as the manager, even though it was rather extraordinary for a seventeen-year-old who was not legally of age to write the bar exam to run a legal office and work independently as a lawyer. One year later, Lowther Pennington Macpherson, John A.'s cousin and a lawyer in Hallowell, Prince Edward County, became gravely ill and left for England to seek treatment. Macpherson asked John A. to move to Hallowell and run his practice for him while he was away. Tragically, Macpherson died at sea on the way home from England, leaving John A. to make a decision about whether or not he wanted to remain a small town lawyer in Hallowell or move back to Kingston where his ambitions would have more room for growth.

Law Society of Upper Canada.
OSGOODE HALL.
—*To wit:*—
DEPOSITED with me this day, pursuant to the standing order of Convocation in that behalf, by Mr. John Alexander McDonald, a Candidate for a Call to the Degree of Barrister at Law of this Society, the amount of the Fee on Call and a Bond to the Society, together with his Petition and Presentation for his Degree.
Treasurer's Office, this 5th *day of* Feby — 1836 } For the TREASURER
Jas. M. Caudelie
Sub Treas.

John A. Macdonald's receipt for application to the Law Society of Upper Canada. (Note the misspelling of Macdonald as McDonald.)

He decided in favour of Kingston and returned to the office of his former employer, George Mackenzie, where misfortune was about to serve Macdonald yet another opportunity. In 1834, a cholera outbreak in Kingston caused the death of nearly three hundred residents, about one tenth of the population. George Mackenzie was amongst those who died, and the result was that John A. became his successor. The following year he opened a new law office on Wellington Street, accepting many of George Mackenzie's former clients. Now twenty years old, he was still a year shy of being able to write the bar exam.

Two weeks after his twenty-first birthday, John A. braved the winter conditions and rough roads and travelled by stagecoach to Toronto in order to sit the exam that would finally give him full status to practise his chosen career. On February 7, 1836, a triumphant John A. Macdonald returned to Kingston, now a fully licensed lawyer and attorney with grand plans for his future.

Meanwhile Hugh Macdonald's mill had finally failed completely. Through family connections, he was offered a position as a clerk in a Kingston bank, and with this in hand, he moved his family back to Kingston and straight

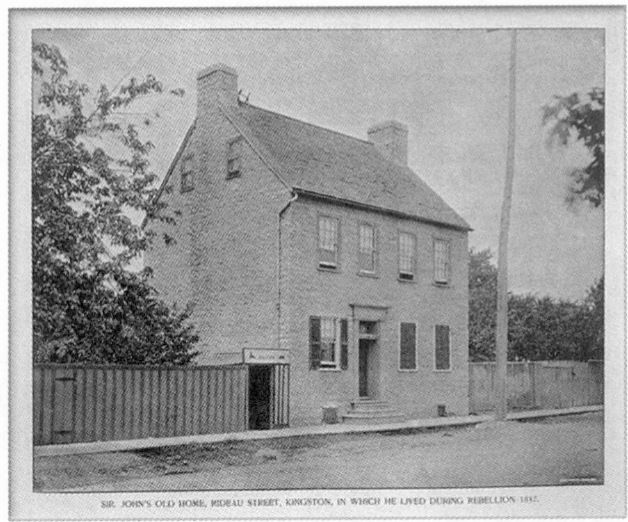

SIR. JOHN'S OLD HOME, RIDEAU STREET, KINGSTON, IN WHICH HE LIVED DURING REBELLION 1837.

John A. Macdonald's stone house on Rideau Street, Kingston *circa* 1835

into John A.'s new and rather substantial limestone house on Rideau Street. In light of his professional status and his income, the young John A. was now the real head of the family.

Although he had first been interested in corporate law, John A. was rapidly becoming attracted to criminal law, perhaps because he saw this as a chance to take on more public and dramatic cases. His first task was to establish a regular roster of clients to bring in steady income and to this end he hired two law students, Alexander Campbell and his old school friend, Oliver Mowat. Between them, they made a living brokering real estate deals, doing title searches, chasing down debtors, and completing various corporate business transactions.

Such a business transaction was the very reason that sixteen-year-old Eliza Grimason sought out and found John A. Macdonald. One of John

A.'s first clients, Eliza needed some legal advice about a property on Division Street that she and her husband were contemplating purchasing. Short, stout, poor, Irish, and uneducated, Eliza Grimason was a force to be reckoned with. Something about her must have tickled John A.'s fancy. Perhaps it was her feisty nature or maybe that in some ways, particularly physically, Eliza resembled his mother, Helen Macdonald. Eliza's appearance at John A.'s office, at a time when businesswomen were almost unheard of, was the beginning of a strange and quite remarkable friendship that endured throughout their lives. Their fifty-five-year relationship has been the subject of much speculation. What is known is that Eliza was one of John A.'s staunchest and richest supporters, giving him both her unconditional, unswerving loyalty and considerable financial support.

For a good part of her life, Eliza owned and managed Grimason House, a popular rough and rowdy Kingston tavern, which still exists and is now known as the Royal Tavern, 344 Princess Street. Eliza and her husband, Henry Grimason, leased the property from John A. in 1856. When Henry died in 1867, John A. never pressed Eliza for the £300 annual rent. In return, Eliza kept two rooms upstairs for John A. and served him dinner and drinks.

Tavern dinners were usually about twenty-five cents. Whiskey cost five cents. Typical tavern dinners of the day consisted of a meat-based main course with vegetables, accompanied by bread and butter, followed by some sort of pudding which might include a slice of cake or pie, or a serving of steamed pudding and custard.

John A., who was a slight man, was never known for his hearty appetite. Left to his own devices, he was apt to forget mealtimes altogether, though it seems he rarely forgot to have a drink. He thrived on companionship, however, and he fully understood that food brought people together. After a night of drinking, John A. often slept upstairs at Grimason House in one of the allocated rooms. According to legend, Eliza would awaken him on

Sunday mornings with tea and toast, in time that he would not be late arriving at church.

Eliza was John A.'s biggest admirer. There is no doubt she loved him—she is on record as having said so publicly on more than one occasion. One election night she walked into a committee room, kissed John A., and then left without saying a word. The only time he ever lost an election, she was at his side saying, "There's not a man like him on the livin' earth." Not only did she contribute financially to his campaigns, but she also bribed voters with free food and free drinks. Most importantly of all, she kept John A.'s confidence. For his part, John A. allowed Eliza to sit in on private political gatherings and included her in a great many events that neither one of his wives was ever privy to. He invited her to visit him in Ottawa and kept a photograph of her alongside his mother's. There's little doubt it was a love affair of sorts, but whether or not it was purely platonic remains a mystery that no longer matters. Eliza Grimason kept John A. well-fed and well-watered—a form of love they both understood. When she died, she was laid to rest in the Cataraqui Cemetery, adjacent to the Macdonald family plot.

THE TWENTY-FIVE-CENT TAVERN DINNER

John A., like many men of his era, spent a large amount of time in the tavern. Taverns were important social gathering places in the nineteenth century. In most towns they were the major meeting place, whether for political gatherings and elections or as a place to discuss business transactions, job opportunities, and crop prices. Taverns were the place where all the news of the day was broadcast. In addition, there was gambling and entertainment, whether legal or not. Drunkenness and violence were commonplace. It wasn't until much later in the 1800s and early 1900s that the temperance movement began to influence the rates of alcohol consumption.

It was not unusual for taverns to be run by women, particularly widowed women for whom very few occupations were possible. They could make a living running a tavern, and it was socially acceptable to do so.

For travellers, taverns were among the few places one could get a meal and a room, especially in smaller towns. As there was no indoor plumbing, rooms had a commode and a washstand with a jug and wash basin. Female travellers in Upper Canada were generally confined to one of the bedrooms or, depending on the size of the tavern, there might be a small dining room where women were allowed to congregate and bring their children. "Gentlewomen" were expected to abstain from drinking alcohol in taverns, though the more daring might have a glass of wine or champagne at a dinner party.

Tavern food was the only food widely available on the road. Roasts, hearty stews, and meat pies were common tavern fare. Stews and pies made good use of a variety of leftover meats. They were tasty, and the meat was tender thanks, in part, to being cooked a second time, often with gravy or butter, and sealed in by either pastry (called at that time "paste") or potatoes, or sometimes both.

The following recipe for medley pie is from *The Canadian Housewife's Manual of Cookery*. It would be typical of many tavern meat pies. The fact that it uses a variety of meats would have made perfect for using up leftovers. Pork and beef were more commonplace than either mutton or lamb, but the British had a particular fondness for lamb.

MEDLEY PIE

Cut slices of beef, mutton, or pork with bacon (or use bacon alone); lay them in a dish with sliced apples and a little onion chopped placed in alternate layers, with the meat. Season with pepper and salt and add a tablespoon of sugar; pour in a little stock, cover with short crust, and bake slowly.

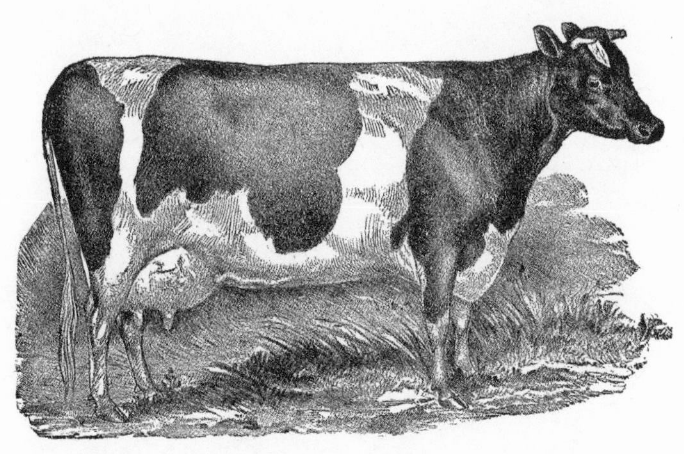

CHAPTER SIX

Rebellion, Courtroom Drama, and a Full English Breakfast

1837–42

Macdonald quickly gained a reputation as an astute and courageous lawyer with a vast knowledge of the law. He believed deeply in the right to a fair trial and the integrity of the legal system. He took on cases which others were loath to defend. For two years, from 1837 to 1839, he took on several controversial and challenging cases, proving his ingenuity and legal prowess, even when he lost.

One of those cases was that of William Brass, who stood accused of raping an eight-year-old girl—a heinous crime for which a guilty verdict meant a death sentence. Macdonald argued that Brass was too drunk to have been capable of committing a sexual act. Ironically, given his own proclivity for consuming alcohol, he also argued that Brass's addiction to alcohol was a form of insanity. Despite these arguments, Brass was found guilty and hanged. Unfortunately his hanging was a harrowing affair, because the rope was too long and he fell to the ground, landing alive in his own coffin, whereupon he began insisting that this proved his innocence. He was hanged again in short order, making him the first but not the only man in Canadian history to be hanged twice. Despite the fact that Macdonald lost the case, the media and the public both seemed to side with Macdonald. There was widespread recognition that a fair and intelligent trial was a necessary part of the justice system.

While Macdonald was building a career in the criminal courtroom, other trouble was developing. Two armed uprisings, known as the Rebellions of 1837, were brewing.

The first rebellion took place in Lower Canada beginning in November 1837. It was fuelled by French animosity toward the governing English elite and led by Louis-Joseph Papineau and the Patriotes, who wanted greater control of civil salaries, economic development at the local level, and better access to government positions by the francophone middle class. English and French groups fought in the streets of Montreal, and fifty-eight Patriotes were killed before British authorities were brought in to quell the uprising.

The second rebellion took place in Upper Canada and was led by William Lyon Mackenzie, grandfather of William Lyon Mackenzie King, who later became prime minister of Canada. Mackenzie and his followers were recent immigrants from Great Britain and did not want to see a perpetuation in Upper Canada of the same concentration of power they had known in England. They set out to seize Toronto, the capital of Upper Canada, with the intention of overthrowing the government and setting up an American-style republic.

Macdonald was in Toronto when Mackenzie gathered the rebel forces at Montgomery's Tavern on Yonge Street.[11] He joined the government side, a force of about a thousand men, who marched up Yonge Street with their muskets and two cannons and flushed the insurgents out of the tavern, ending the Siege at Toronto with what was essentially an overblown skirmish. After this defeat, Mackenzie fled to the United States, where he lived in exile.

It was the only time in Macdonald's life that he bore arms. Later he told his private secretary, Joseph Pope, "The day was hot, my feet were blistered—I was but a weary boy—and I thought I should have dropped under the weight of the old flint musket, which galled my shoulder. But I managed to keep up with my companion, a grim old soldier who seemed impervious to fatigue."[12]

In Kingston, eight of Mackenzie's loyal supporters assembled with weapons, prepared to fight a battle of their own. But when nobody else joined them, the men gave up their cause and returned home, or more likely back to a tavern. When the eight men were accused of treason for taking up arms against the Queen, John A. Macdonald successfully defended them, despite the fact that he himself had fought on the other side of the rebellion.

The rebellions were important because they helped pave the way to the first British North America Act of 1840, which saw Upper and Lower Canada united as the new Province of Canada in 1841. This led to the act which established the Dominion of Canada: the British North America Act of 1867. So although the rebel leaders, Papineau and Mackenzie, were unsuccessful in their attempts to overthrow the government, their actions had a lasting impact on the future of the country.

Back in his law practice, after taking part in the rebellion in Toronto, Macdonald continued to take on notorious, unpopular, and difficult cases. In the Battle at Prescott in 1839, he helped a group of American invaders who were seeking to "liberate" Upper Canada from British oppression. The invaders, foreign nationals, were to be tried in a military court-martial and as such were not privy to a civilian defence lawyer. Macdonald recognized the injustice of the situation, and he tried to advise the men on a defence strategy. Nevertheless, the eight were found guilty.

In the same year John A. Macdonald made his last appearance as a criminal lawyer, defending Brandt Brandt, a member of the Mohawk nation who was accused of murder. Again, Macdonald argued that the drunkenness of everyone involved cast reasonable doubt on what had actually happened. His defence was plausible and the jury agreed. Brandt was found guilty of manslaughter instead of murder, and he was sentenced to a six months' jail term.

As a criminal lawyer, Macdonald had acquired a strong reputation, and he had the respect of the newspapers. Although the public was not always on his side, they certainly knew who he was. Nevertheless, in 1839, Macdonald decided it was time to change direction and make some serious money by refocussing his practice on commercial law, taking on the directorships of several companies. He began buying real estate—a sideline that he kept up his entire life, although he rarely made any profit. He had a knack for buying high and selling low, more often than not losing money on the properties that he bought in fits of giddy speculation.

In 1841, fifty-nine-year-old Hugh Macdonald died, leaving John A. with full financial responsibility for his mother and unmarried sisters. He was just twenty-six years old, single, and for a young man who was already working hard as a lawyer, the additional responsibility seems to have been a tipping point. He fell ill, such that he was scarcely able to work. John A. complained of stomach pains and at one point collapsed to the ground. He was prescribed morphine for pain, but his condition remained undiagnosed. Eventually, on his doctor's advice, he began planning a trip to England in the hope that by distancing himself from his work and his woes, his health would improve.

In January 1842, Macdonald spent three dizzy nights gambling in a high-stakes game known as loo. He won two thousand pounds, a windfall that he knew he would never be able to repeat and one that made him vow to never gamble again. He left almost immediately for Britain, sailing from Boston. He was away for six months, and during that time not only did he fall in love with England, but he also made the acquaintance of his cousin Isabella, and whether it was her British manners and customs that charmed him, or whether he truly fell in love with her, he invited her to come to Canada the following year.

There was no doubt about Macdonald's feelings for England. He was smitten. In London he spent his time going to parliamentary debates, as well as dining, drinking, and shopping. He visited Oxford, Cambridge, and Windsor, where he was able to arrange an invitation for a private viewing of Queen Victoria's apartments. He toured the Lake District and spent time in both Manchester and Chester. He visited family members in Scotland and

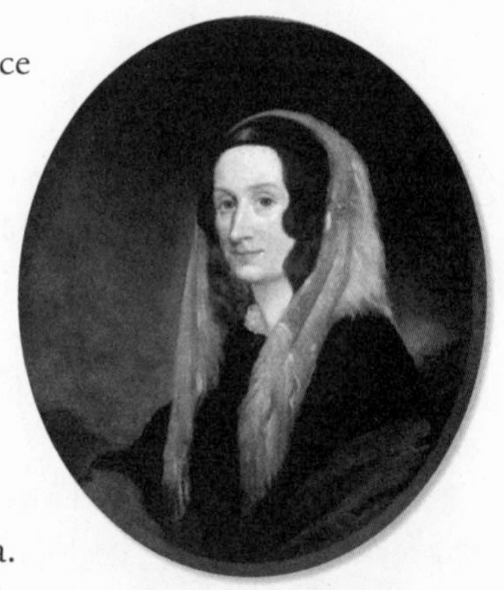
Isabella Clark

the Isle of Man. He had a grand time, since his winnings from loo enabled him to go on a spending spree, purchasing all manner of things, including a great many books, luxurious fabrics, kitchen and household items, chimney ornaments, and fashionable clothing. It was a most extraordinarily lively convalescence.

His letters home to his mother could scarcely contain his newfound anglophilia. Amongst other things, he wrote to tell her at some length about how well he was eating and seemed particularly delighted with his breakfast. He wrote:

> *You would be surprised at the breakfasts I eat. Wilson* [his travelling companion, Thomas Wilson, a representative of the Commercial Bank in Montreal] *laughs as he sees roll after roll disappear & eggs & bacon after roll. My dinners are equally satisfactory to myself... Only fancy, my commencing my dinner with a sole fried, with shrimp sauce, demolishing a large steak, and polishing off with bread & cheese and a quart of London Stout.*[13]

Between the food, the socializing, and the shopping spree, by late summer a fully convalesced John A. returned to Kingston with his treasure trove of gifts and goods, a renewed enthusiasm for his life and work, and for better or worse, the promise of an upcoming visit from his cousin, Isabella.

THE FULL ENGLISH BREAKFAST: CANADIAN STYLE

The breakfasts John A. experienced in England were not typical in the colonies. London at the time of his visit was the wealthiest city in the world, and the British Empire was at the pinnacle of its power. The English had access to commodities from around the globe, and the gentry and upper classes, in particular, enjoyed a lifestyle that could not be replicated in Upper or Lower Canada.

The Victorians believed breakfast was the most important meal of the day for reasons of both health and civility. The wealthy upper classes might eat a breakfast with several different types of meat, including bacon, black pudding (sausage made from blood), pork sausages, game, and fish, as well as stewed fruit, eggs, beans, tomato, mushrooms, toast, and crumpets, all accompanied by pots of tea.

In North America, records and early cookbooks focus on breakfasts that were mostly grains in various forms, such as oatmeal, bread, pancakes, fritters, and cornbread, often known as johnny cake or Indian bread. Cornbread was a remarkably popular staple.

While eggs, bacon, sausages, steaks, and salt pork were all available and all appeared at least occasionally on breakfast tables, in general, the expansive full-English breakfast was certainly not the norm for most settlers. Eggs were a vital source of protein in the diet, and it was not unusual for homeowners, even in town, to keep chickens. There are several mentions in the letters and diaries of the Macdonald family of keeping poultry, and while eggs would have been regularly on the menu, there are few references in early North American literature to eggs being served for breakfast. Until well into the mid-1800s, eggs were primarily used for baking and served at lunch, dinner, or supper.

Cornbread, however, was served routinely for breakfast. Early settlers in North America were introduced to cornmeal by the indigenous people, and settlers referred to it as Indian meal. Most early cookbooks contain several recipes for Indian pudding or Indian bread, which also came to be called corn pone (pone from the Algonquin word "apan," meaning baked), and johnny bread as it is still sometimes known today.

Cornmeal was used to make cakes, breads, muffins, pancakes, and porridge. Without it, settlers would have scarcely survived the first harsh years in the New World. It was a staple part of the diet until well into the 1900s and continues to be so, though perhaps more in the United States and Mexico than in Canada, where settlement of the prairies increased the availability of some of the finest wheat in the world.

Cornbread is a versatile dish that can be served as a stand-alone item with butter, maple syrup, jam, or honey. It can also be served alongside eggs, beans, bacon, sausages, soup or stew. All early North American cookbooks contained recipes for cornbread. *The Cook Not Mad* lists four different cornbread recipes. The first is called "A tasty Indian Pudding." The next two are both entitled, "Another." A fourth is entitled "Johnny Cake or hoe cake." The recipe included here is from *The Canadian Home Cook Book* (1887) and was chosen over the others because of its superior flavour and texture, due to the addition of baking soda.

JOHNNIE CAKE

One pint of corn meal, one teacup of flour, two eggs, one pint of sweet milk, one tablespoon of molasses, one tablespoon of melted butter, a little salt, one teaspoon of soda, one teaspoon of cream of tartar; bake in square tins.

258512

Kingston, September 1st 1843.

John Alexander Macdonald and Isabella Clark, both of Kingston, were, by Licence from His Excellency, The Right Honorable Sir Charles Theophilus Metcalfe Bart. G.C.B. Governor General of British North America &c. &c. &c. married by me, on this first day of September, One Thousand Eight Hundred and Forty-three

Thos. Wilson
Charles Stuart } Witnesses

John Machar
Minr. of St. Andrews Church

Extracted from the Marriage Register of Saint Andrews Church, Kingston, on this first day of September, One Thousand Eight Hundred and Forty-three

John Machar Minr.

John A. Macdonald and Isabella Clark's marriage licence

CHAPTER SEVEN

Political Ambitions and a Wedding Cake

1843

Fully recovered from his mysterious illness and all fired up by his travels to England, John A. returned to Kingston with a renewed spirit. Attending the British parliamentary debates had planted fertile ideas in his head, and one of the first things he did was to ask his friends for advice on what one would do to prepare for a career in political office. Their recommendation was to join the Protestant fraternal organization known as the Orange Lodge and to consider running to become an alderman.

He did just that, and to cover all the bases, he became a Mason as well. Shortly after, in early 1843, John A. Macdonald announced his intention to run as a candidate for the position of alderman for the City of Kingston. The public attention he had earned while he was a criminal lawyer gave him a head start, but his victory was far from certain. Macdonald's Irish opponent, Colonel Jackson, fought a feisty and spirited battle. Macdonald campaigned vigorously and went so far as to take the unusual step of purchasing newspaper advertisements, promising that nothing would stand in the way of honouring his commitment to fulfill the duties imposed on him by the position of alderman.

Five days before the election, Macdonald held an elegant soiree at his Brock Street home for the new governor general, Sir Charles Metcalfe, a wealthy peer, born in India, whose career included tours of duty as the governor of Agra, acting governor general of India, governor of the Northwest Territories, and governor of Jamaica. The fact that Macdonald could host and hold his own in such elegant company speaks volumes about both his political aptitude and his bravado.

On March 28, Macdonald won a seat on Kingston's city council. His supporters carried him from the tavern and into the street atop a chair. Moments later, he was dumped unceremoniously onto the street, into the slush and manure. Picking himself up amongst the throngs of bystanders and drunken revellers, Macdonald brushed himself off, turned to the revellers and said, "Isn't it strange that I should have downfall so soon?"[14] The crowd roared with laughter.

In early summer, his cousin Isabella arrived in Kingston from England. Before long, Macdonald was courting her. Some descriptions of Isabella show her as a scheming woman set on marriage to her cousin; others portray her as sweet, frail, and child-like. She was, however, refined and morally upright—a gentlewoman—and marriage to her would ensure Macdonald's credentials as a gentleman. The date was set for September, just a few months after her arrival. Although John A. was known for being drawn to women of questionable moral character and was on record as having told his subordinates, "There's no wisdom below the belt,"[15] he was smart enough to know that he needed Isabella in his life.

They were united in holy matrimony at St. Andrew's Church in Kingston on September 1, 1843. The Reverend John Machar presided over the ceremony, and Charles Stuart, John A.'s school friend, acted as best man. The couple and the family were home by lunch time and celebrated with a drink and a slice of wedding cake—considered among the most important rituals of any wedding ceremony in the era.

In his biography of his uncle, James Pennington Macpherson paints a sweet picture of the early domestic harmony enjoyed by John A. and Isabella. He was encouraged to go often to their home.

This house, situated on Brock Street, was large and commodious and contained all the comforts and conveniences then known to Canadian civilization. There was also a fine carriage and a pair of horses, Mohawk and Charlie, Macpherson wrote.

> *I spent some of the happiest days of my life, being allowed the honour of sitting beside the coachman if the carriage was taken out, or at other times, the almost equally enjoyable privilege of being my uncle's companion in his library. We seldom talked; he was deep in his books, while I had a corner to myself where were garnered together.... King Arthur and His Knights at the Round Table, The Arabian Nights Entertainment, etc. etc. I have no doubt but that I was troublesome, but I cannot recollect ever receiving from him one unkind word. On the contrary, I was always made happy by a warm greeting, a pleasant smile, an encouraging word, or an affectionate pat on the head. Often I used to meet him on the street, when going to or from school, and then it was his delight to indulge in the pleasant fiction that he was my debtor to an unknown amount, and proceed to liquidate this debt to the extent of the half-pence he might have in his pocket.... I came to regard him as the most generous man I had ever known.*[16]

The young Macpherson was equally enamoured of Isabella and in his memoir reminisced about her "sweet gentleness of manner and tender sympathetic nature."

So despite any strategic reasons that John A. and Isabella each had for marrying, it seemed an idyllic relationship, and it was not long before John A. had a chance to use his newfound respectability to advance his career.

WEDDINGS IN THE 1800s

British and North American weddings in the first half of the 1800s were relatively simple, pragmatic affairs. Brides generally had few clothes and were married in their best dress, which could be a silk dress if they had one, almost always coloured or even black. It was Queen Victoria's marriage to Prince Albert on February 10, 1840, in a splendid white satin dress that paved the way to the modern white wedding. The changes, however, were slow in coming to the colonies, as it took time for fashions, fabrics, and patterns to reach the New World. It wasn't until the late 1800s that white weddings became commonplace in Canada, and even then, as a white dress was difficult to clean and maintain, they were not universally accepted.

Weddings in the nineteenth century, though celebratory, were quite sedate, private affairs in part because suitable public halls were largely non-existent. Funerals were on a larger scale because more people were likely to be affected by a death than by a marriage.

John A. and Isabella married at ten o'clock in the morning and returned to the family home for lunch, a toast to their future, and the wedding cake. Their guests would have included family members, the witnesses, a couple of close friends, and very likely the minister, Dr. Machar. The house would have been scrubbed clean and tidied, and the parlour would have been opened up for the event and decorated with fresh flowers.

Like all newly married couples of the era, John A. and Isabella were expected to remain home after their wedding so that well-wishers could drop in and pay their regards, and sample a piece of wedding cake, the traditional symbol of fertility and abundance.

This wedding cake is from *The Canadian Housewife's Manual of Cookery*, 1861.

A WEDDING CAKE

Take one pound of flour, one pound of sifted sugar, two and a half pounds of currants, washed clean, picked and dried, candied citron, orange, lemon-peel, two ounces of each, all cut very fine, a quarter pound of sweet almonds, cut into quarters the long way, a table-spoonful of mixed spice; add all these with the flour, sugar, rub them with your hand til well mixed. Put one pound of butter into a pan and beat into a cream, it should be done with a hand and not with a spoon. After which break the eggs into a basin and beat them up with a whisk and put them into the butter a little at a time. When you add the egg to the butter beat it up until well mixed, then put in the flour, sugar, etc., and about two glasses of brandy. Mix all well together. Have the cake hoop or tin ready, lined with paper, then put in the oven which should not be too hot, but of a good steady heat. To know when sufficiently done, try with a clean knife. Leave it in the mould till the next day. If for a large cake, use double the quantities.

CHAPTER EIGHT

Sex in the City

1844–47

No sooner had John A. and Isabella settled into married life than the government, under the leadership of Robert Baldwin, voted to transfer the capital of the Province of Canada away from Kingston to Montreal. Baldwin was on record as having called Kingston an "Orange hole," referring to the Orange Order, the fraternal Protestant organization dedicated to Protestant supremacy. Macdonald objected and led a protest against the move to Montreal.

By 1844, an election was called and Macdonald stood as the Conservative candidate for Kingston. His platform was practical: build a road from Kingston to the growing lumber village of Bytown (later to become known as Ottawa), settle the neglected rural and back townships, and develop resources. The campaigning was intense and fuelled by alcohol. At twenty-five cents a gallon, the whiskey flowed as freely as the fists flew amongst the voters. On the voting days, October 14 and 15, 1844, the voters did not vote by secret ballots but by shouting aloud their selections.

Macdonald crushed his opponent, Anthony Manahan, winning the election by 275 to 42. He was now part of a Conservative minority government. In November, as Macdonald left to take up his duties as a member of Parliament, Isabella was at home in bed while his mother and his sister waved goodbye from the wharf in Kingston. He left his former law student turned partner, Alexander Campbell, to run the law office, and his wife, Isabella, to run the household. In Montreal, he lived in a boarding house over a grocery store at the corner of St. Maurice and St. Henry Streets.

Just twenty-nine years old John A. Macdonald had everything he had wished for—a lovely home, a successful law business, a wife, a promising career in politics, and the freedom to live alone, learning the ropes of his new position as a backbencher by day and exploring Montreal's gas-lit streets and lively taverns by night. Meanwhile, Macdonald was slowly and surely gaining confidence in his new career as a politician. Initially he was content to be an observer, but by 1845 he had found his voice, speaking out on a number of issues and honing his debating skills.

While Macdonald was away for weeks at a time in Montreal, poor Isabella was adjusting to life in Canada and to sharing a home with her husband's family. Unlike John A., she was not having a good time at all. She suffered from an illness that left her plagued with aches and pains and debilitating weakness. It took a long time before she was diagnosed with a somatization disorder, a condition whereby physical symptoms result from psychiatric conditions, such as anxiety or depression.

Eventually Isabella began taking laudanum (a tincture of opium and alcohol) to numb the pain, and as a result, she immediately developed an opium addiction. In a letter dated June 1845, to her sister Margaret Greene, who had inherited the ancestral estate of her late husband's family in Savannah, Georgia, Isabella wrote, "my head is very confused & I am not sure what to say...."[17]

One month later, John A. also wrote to his sister-in-law, Margaret Greene,

> *My Dear Sister,*
>
> *On this day last year, we left Kingston for New York but I fear it will be sometime before we can hope to do so this year. Isabella has been ill—very ill—with one of her severest attacks. She is*

> *just now recovering and I hope has thrown off for the time her terrible disease. Still, this is not certain, and at all events it has left her in the usual state of prostration that follows every attack.*[18]

He wrote again the following day, to tell her that he had called for the doctor, who was unable to relieve her and thought Isabella in the most precarious state. He signed his letter with the following, "God bless & protect both of you my beloved sisters and enable you to meet the impending anguish with fortitude & resignation. John A. Macdonald."[19]

By July 18, 1845, the couple managed to set off for Savannah, where John A. hoped Isabella might spend the winter. They travelled by boat and train and then by steamboat. Isabella was terribly sick, and at one point John A. thought she might die upon the dock. He wrote to tell Margaret Greene, "The weather was so stormy that all our party were sick, Isabella dreadfully so, and yet strange to say her health and strength seemed to return to her." A few days later he wrote to Margaret again, saying that Isabella was taking opium but walking and eating well. After a particularly bad night in a dirty and bug-ridden hotel room, John A. wrote to tell his sister-in-law, "She bore it like a Shero as she is."[20]

By November the couple had finally reached their destination, whereupon John A. promptly returned to Canada to attend to his political duties and resume his bachelor life in Montreal. One year and one month later, at Christmas, they met up in New York City for a holiday, before they both returned to their separate lives—John A. in Montreal and Isabella in Savannah, with her sister.

Shortly after their New York vacation, Isabella announced that she was expecting a baby. Fearful that she was too ill to withstand pregnancy, John A. made arrangements to move Isabella to New York City, where she would have the best possible medical care. He considered retiring from politics but was determined to give it one last hurrah. To his great surprise, he was appointed to the Cabinet as the receiver general. This was an interesting choice of portfolio for a man who had difficulty managing his own finances.

Macdonald's appointment to the Cabinet attracted the attention of Toronto's *Globe* newspaper, later to become the *Globe and Mail*, which promptly dismissed him as "harmless."[21] George Brown, the *Globe*'s founder, eventually became a fierce critic and political rival of Macdonald's.

Despite his new responsibilities, John A. was with Isabella in New York City when she gave birth on August 2, 1847. Isabella laboured for thirty-seven hours and was one of the first women ever to receive anaesthesia during childbirth. Finally, with the aid of forceps, she delivered a baby boy. They named him John Alexander. He had his father's astonishing nose and his lanky physique. The entire family rejoiced at the birth of a vigorous baby. That ailing thirty-seven-year-old Isabella had delivered a healthy child and survived childbirth was nothing short of a miracle. Isabella's sister, Maria Macpherson, soon whisked the baby away to Kingston to be cared for by a wet nurse.

John A. was ecstatic about the birth of his son. Even so, within a month, he left a frail and recuperating Isabella in New York City and returned to Montreal to take up his role in the Cabinet amidst an unstable political climate. The Conservative party was under fire, and the government looked set to dissolve. The economy was depressed, and there was a great deal of social unrest. An election was called for the period of late December 1847 into early January 1848. Macdonald retained his Kingston seat with an easy victory, but elsewhere the Conservatives were soundly defeated and resigned office in March 1848. A new Liberal government was formed.

Meanwhile John A. was burdened with a litany of problems. First, his mother, Helen Macdonald, suffered a series of strokes and required constant care. Then his law partner, Alexander Campbell, was balking at having to carry all the work in the law practice and receiving only a small share of the profits. Finally John A.'s finances were teetering precariously towards disaster, having been severely depleted by Isabella's medical costs. Worried about his wife, his mother, his law practice, his finances, the state of the nation and missing his baby son, John A. sought refuge in the lounges and smoking rooms and taverns of Montreal.

THE FRENCH INFLUENCE

Macdonald, influenced by his time in Montreal, had become a passionate advocate for a united Canada that included both English and French interests. He once famously said, "Let us be English or let us be French... but above all let us be Canadians." He believed the similarities between the two outweighed the differences, and he also believed that French and English Canadians had more in common with each other than they did with Americans.

In fact, the Scottish and the French shared many similarities, one of which was the love of food and alcohol. Macdonald, whose drinking preferences ran to champagne, claret, and brandy rather than whiskey, found himself quite at home in Montreal's taverns. Here he was introduced to tourtière, the classic French Canadian meat pie that bore a strong resemblance to both Scotch pie, which was often but not always filled with ground mutton, and the English Melton Mowbray pie, filled with ground or chopped jellied pork.

The history of tourtière is the subject of some debate and a great many culinary history essays. The name appears to be derived from a cooking vessel of the same name that was originally used to bake a variety of meat and seafood pies. Eventually the pies themselves became known by the name of the vessel. Some culinary historians believe the pie was called a tourtière because it was originally made with passenger pigeons, known in French as *les tourtes*.

Regardless, tourtière, a French-Canadian tradition, has been mentioned in the literature since about 1611, and it is widely regarded as a significant contribution to Canada's culinary repertoire.

Tourtières are often made with ground pork, beef or veal, and sometimes a combination of these three. Other variations are made with fish, venison, duck, rabbit, or other wild game. The classic Montreal tourtière, made with finely ground pork, is probably the closest companion to the British meat pies that Macdonald was most familiar with.

The version here is from an old Montreal family recipe, courtesy of Kingston writer and historian David More. A glass of Macdonald's favourite drop, a good claret, is a perfect companion. And some caramelized onion confit would not go amiss, either.

A CLASSIC MONTREAL TOURTIÈRE

Pastry for a 9 inch double crust pie
1 pound lean ground pork
1/2 pound regular ground beef
1 onion, finely diced
1 clove garlic, minced
1/2 cup water
1 1/2 teaspoons salt
2 teaspoons fresh thyme, chopped or 1 tsp dried thyme, crushed
1/2 teaspoon ground sage
freshly ground black pepper
1/4 teaspoon ground nutmeg

Preheat oven to 425 degrees F (220 degrees C).

Roll out pastry and place bottom crust in pie plate.

In a frypan sauté the pork, beef, onion, and garlic. When the meat is lightly browned, add water, salt, thyme, sage, black pepper and nutmeg. Cook over medium heat until mixture boils; stirring occasionally. Reduce heat to low and simmer until meat is cooked, about 5 minutes.

Spoon the meat mixture into the pie crust and top with remaining rolled prepared pastry. Pinch pastry edges to seal. Cut several vents in top crust so steam can escape.

Cover edges of pie with strips of aluminum foil to prevent over-cooking.

Bake in preheated oven for 20 minutes, remove foil and return to oven. Bake for an additional 15 to 20 minutes or until pie is golden brown. Let cool 10 minutes before serving.

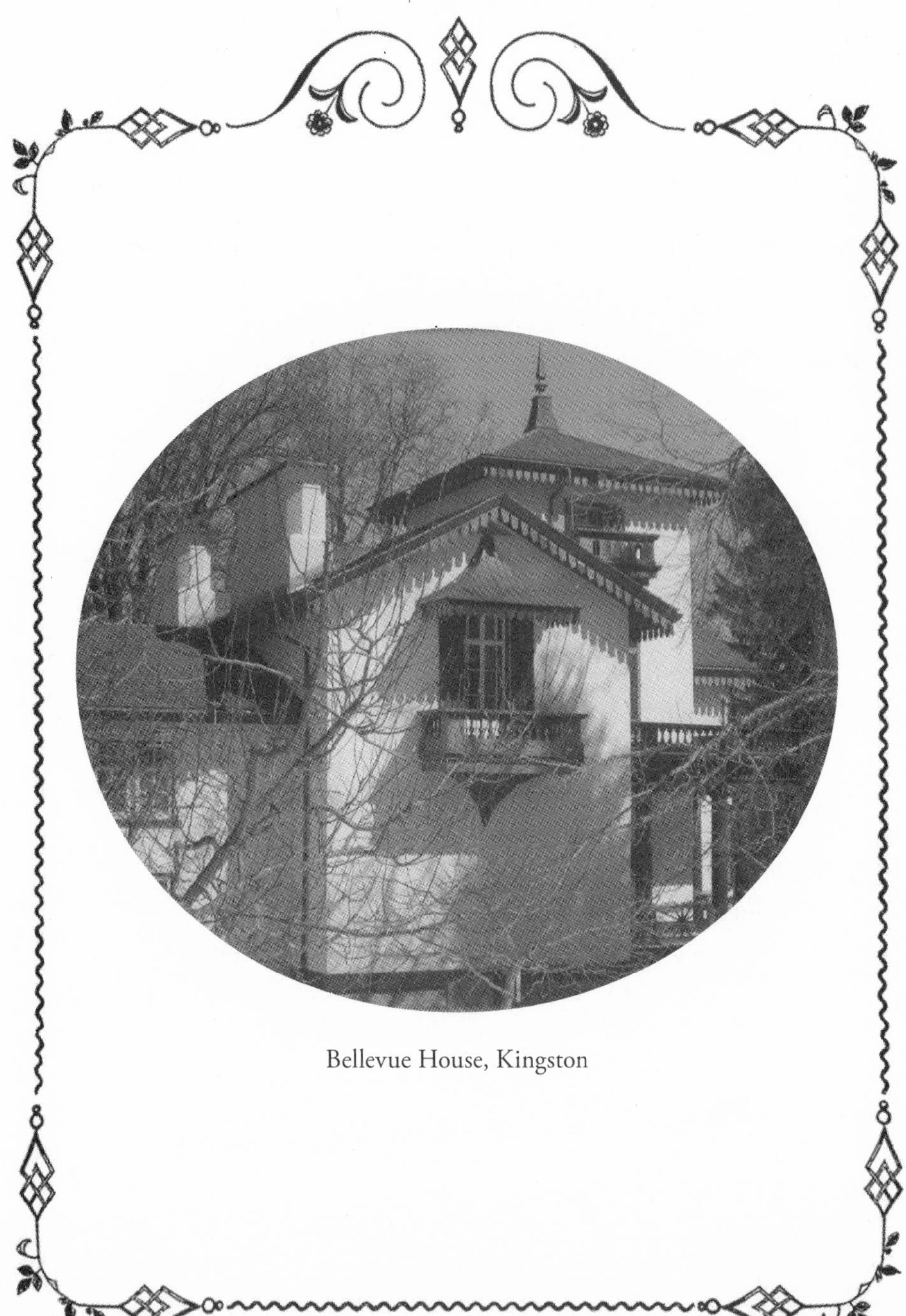

Bellevue House, Kingston

CHAPTER NINE

The Burning of the Houses of Parliament

1848–50

Isabella remained in New York City for a year, finally returning to Canada in late summer 1848. In the meantime John A. had organized to rent a Tuscan-style villa near the shore of Lake Ontario in Kingston in the hope that the change of location and a spacious house near the water might be good for Isabella's health. The villa, Bellevue House, now a national historic site, was built by a man who made his fortune as a grocer and who may have had more money than taste.

In a letter to his sister Margaret in August 1848, John A. wrote,

> *I have taken a cottage or rather, I beg its pardon, a Villa.... It is a large roomy house where I hope to see you and Jane next spring. The house was built for a retired grocer, who was resolved to have an "Eyetalian Willar," and has built the most fantastic concern imaginable....*
>
> *P.S. A propos of my landlord—here is a conundrum for Jane. Why is mixing wine or adulterating sugar a more heinous crime than murder? ANS. Because murder is a gross offence but adulterating sugar is a grocer offence.*[22]

Despite her new home, Isabella remained unwell and had now developed a cough that produced blood, which was a possible sign of tuberculosis. She stayed in her bed but managed, nevertheless, to forcibly rule the house. John A. wrote in one his letters that both family and staff began to refer to her as "the Invisible Lady," whose orders must be followed.

On September 21, 1848, mere months after the Macdonald family had moved into their new home, tragedy struck. The nurse went into baby John's room and found him dead in his cot. Just thirteen months old and only recently reacquainted with his mother, his cause of death was listed as convulsions. He was buried soon after beside his grandfather, Hugh Macdonald, in a Kingston cemetery. It was a dramatic turning point in John A. and Isabella's lives. The tragedy changed them forever. She turned to opium; he focussed all his attention on his career and found solace in his drinking.

In February 1849, John A. returned to Montreal for a new session of Parliament. The Liberal government proposed a Rebellion Losses Bill that would see ninety thousand pounds, a very large sum of government funds, compensate those who had suffered in Lower Canada in the rebellions of 1837 and 1838. The Tories felt the bill was essentially a reward for treason. At one point the proceedings became so intensely heated that John A. sent a note to William Hume Blake, the Liberal solicitor general for Canada West, inviting him to a duel. It was not the first time John A. had been part of a challenge to a duel in the House of Commons, although it was the first time he had made the request himself. Both men left the house, pursued by the sergeant-at-arms. John A. was quickly apprehended, but Blake appeared to be in hiding. Before the night was out, the police held both men in custody and released them only after a reluctant John A. withdrew his invitation.

The vote on the Rebellion Losses Bill took place on February 22, 1849. John A., using the only tactic available to him, spoke until late in the day, opposing the bill. He was powerless to do anything further and the bill passed the House.

Not long after this, John A. applied for a leave of absence to attend to urgent but unspecified private business. His request was approved, and he was back home in Kingston when Montreal's right-wing Conservative anglophone population burned down the Parliament Buildings and threatened to seek annexation with the United States. The Conservatives were in complete disarray, and since John A. despaired of the attitudes and actions of some of his colleagues, he moved quickly to disassociate himself. He began by helping to organize the British North American League, which condemned both violence and annexation.

With the Parliament Buildings in ashes, once again the location of Canada's capital was up for consideration. It was decided that the capital should alternate between Quebec City and Toronto every five years. Macdonald disagreed. He believed that Canada needed a permanent capital and that it should be Kingston. He rallied the league and organized a political convention in Kingston in July 1849. He managed to get 150 delegates to Kingston, although he appeared to have little to say, provoking *The Globe* to write, "He never says much anywhere except in barrooms."

John A. was soon distracted by other remarkable news. Isabella was pregnant again. In the mid-1800s it was almost unheard of for a forty-year-old woman, let alone a very ill and opium addicted 40-year-old, to become pregnant. In his 1986 essay, James McSherry wrote the following about Isabella Macdonald:

> Her illness had far reaching effects on John, for, in the words of a biographer, "he had become a family man whose home was a hotel or a lodging house; a bachelor husband who had to go for companionship to bars and lounges and smoking

> rooms; a frustrated host who drank too much on occasion; partly because it was the only way he could entertain, and because it passed the empty time, and because it was an easy way to forget."
>
> What ailed Isabella? What was this disease that rendered Isabella Macdonald such a hopeless invalid and yet allowed her to conceive twice and carry both pregnancies to term?
>
> What ailed Isabella? Retrospective diagnosis is fraught with difficulty, but the probabilities are that Isabella had pulmonary tuberculosis, a hysterical personality, complicated migraine and opiate dependence. One can only wonder at John A. Macdonald's patience and kindness, for life with Isabella must have been a sore trial.[23]

Almost immediately upon learning that Isabella was pregnant again, John A. received the devastating news that Alexander Campbell had decided to withdraw from the law office because he was no longer able to cope with Macdonald's absences and the burden of overwork. Macdonald tried to draw up a new contract, but Campbell told him bluntly, "I feel I have been doing too much and getting too little." Harsh words perhaps, but Macdonald had been leaning hard on Campbell for a long time. The final straw for Campbell was that the company was in debt to the tune of eighteen hundred pounds while John A. kept spending money hand over fist.

John A. bought Campbell out and moved the office to 343 King Street East, Kingston. The site is now a pub called Sir John's Public House. Meanwhile Macdonald mortgaged the Brock Street house, where his mother and sisters lived, and moved Isabella and her collection of servants into 180 Johnson Street.

For a short time, things seemed stable. Then on November 13, Isabella's thirty-seven-year-old sister, Jane, died in Georgia. Isabella took the news

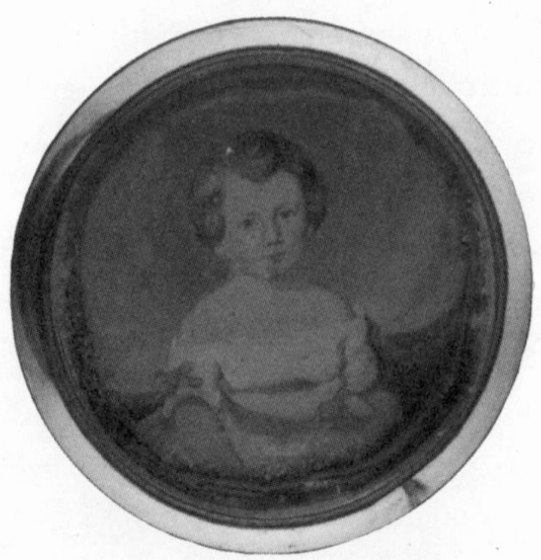

Locket with copy of a painting of Hugh John Macdonald
by William Sawyer, 1852

hard and began suffering premature contractions. For the next four months Isabella was confined to bed, awaiting the birth of her child. Finally, early the following spring, she gave birth to another healthy baby boy. John A. recorded the details of the birth as follows, "Wednesday, March 13, 1850—My darling Isa has a fine boy. Saturday, June 1—Darling baby christened by Dr. Machar, Hugh John Macdonald."[24]

Hugh John's birth was a happy interlude in an otherwise difficult time. Not long after he was born, Helen Macdonald suffered another stroke, and John A. learned that one of his dearest long-term friends and his best man, Charles Stuart, was deathly ill with consumption. Unmotivated as a back bencher, he did not return to the legislature, now sitting in Toronto, for several months. Meanwhile he divided his time between his law office, his family, and his dying friend. Once back in the political arena, he focussed his energies on trying to persuade the assembly to exempt trust and loan companies from present usury laws in order that they could charge higher interest rates. The legislation passed with barely a notice, thereby saving the British-owned

Trust and Loan Company of Upper Canada, one of Macdonald's biggest legal clients, from certain bankruptcy, and thus saving Macdonald himself from the same fate.

During this time, John A. received an urgent summons to return to Kingston where Isabella had taken a turn for the worse and was scarcely able to lift her hand to her head. He provided comfort to her and took care of finding a new nurse for Hugh John, but the really urgent matter was for him to find a way to strengthen his own finances for the future and for the upkeep of his extended family. Never one to think small, a broke John A. set sail, in a first-class cabin, for London, England, where his plan was to raise investment funds for the Kingston branch of the Trust and Loan Company. Although the details are scant, it appears that his efforts were successful. Between champagne and caviar receptions, he managed to raise half a million pounds of investment funding. He returned to Canada in the late fall. His relationships in England were reaffirmed, his financial situation was more secure, and his taste for fine food and high society had been temporarily sated. Although he enjoyed social events, Macdonald was equally fond of a quiet family dinner at home or drinks in the tavern, catching up on local news.

FAMILY DINNERS IN UPPER CANADA

Late autumn was a time of plenty in Upper Canada in the mid-1800s. Throughout summer and fall, all manner of fruit, vegetables, fish, and meat had been harvested and set up for storage by being either jellied, dried, smoked, salted, pickled, or buried. Every means possible were used to prepare food for the long, hard winters endured by settlers. Winter poverty was a reality for many, particularly in rural areas where paid work all but stopped in the winter months. In addition to securing enough food, there were coal and firewood to be laid in. Poor planning for winters could have disastrous consequences. There were reports of children freezing to their deaths inside their own homes, and depending on the winter, food supplies had often dwindled to almost nothing by spring when sickness, malnutrition, and starvation were all harsh realities. Though the wealthy might have had the means to enjoy winter with skating and tobogganing and mulled wine, all settlers needed to plan carefully to stock their pantries and larders before the onset of winter.

Mushrooms, peas, beans, strawberries, cherries, quinces, crab apples, squash, and pumpkins were dried in the sun. Blueberries and other berries, chokecherries, grapes, plums, gooseberries, and currants were made into jellies, preserves, and wine. Cucumbers and cabbage were preserved in brine in stone crocks. Apples were dried or barrelled or made into cider. Cabbages, potatoes, and turnips were buried in the ground to prevent freezing. Onions, carrots, and beets were stored in sawdust in wooden bins. Chestnuts and whatever other nuts were available were harvested and dried briefly in the sun. Sage and thyme and rosemary were hung in bunches. Honey and maple syrup were stored in jars and crocks. Eggs were preserved in various ways, including being stored in lime water or packed in salt; the salt could be used over as the eggs were used. Fish were dried and salted. Animals fattened all summer were butchered. Sausage meat was stuffed into homemade sack cloth casings or packed in stone crocks. Large barrels or crocks of pork or ham were cured in brine or salted down. The most popular preserved meat was pork. Sausages, pickled hams, salt pork, and smoked bacon were all commonplace.

Yorkshire-born artist and gentlewoman Anne Langton moved to Upper Canada in 1837. In her letters and journals she recorded many details of her daily life, including this menu for a typical dinner party given in 1839: "Perhaps you would like to know what we gave them for dinner. Soup, boiled pork (the national dish), stewed goose, and chicken pie, with vegetables. Second course—plum pudding, apple tart, and a trifle."[25]

Sausages were immensely popular fare, in particular pork sausages which were a great favourite of the British. When a pig was butchered, the leftover bits of meat were made into sausages which were then packed into crocks and covered in hot, rendered fat. As the fat cooled it sealed and the sausages kept surprisingly well. They were used in toad in the hole, a dish that was greatly favoured by children, in part because of its name. The British had a penchant for comically named dishes such as bubble and squeak, jam roly poly, and spotted dick, a plain steamed pudding "spotted" with raisins—all of which seemed to appeal to the young and the young at heart.

Toad in the hole is a casserole of sausages cooked in a Yorkshire pudding batter. One of the first references to toad in the hole comes from the Oxford English Dictionary who recorded the phrase in 1787. Mrs. Beeton included a version in her 1861 cookbook. This version below is from the *Fiskin Manuscript Cookbook*. It is particularly good served with brown onion gravy.

The remarkably simple gooseberry pie recipe that follows comes from Mrs. Nourse's *Modern Practical Cookery, Pastry, Confectionery, Pickling and Preserving: With a Great Variety of Useful and Economical Receipts*. Mrs. Elizabeth Nourse ran a small culinary arts school in Edinburgh and played an important part in Canadian culinary history when her comprehensive 464-page cookbook was published in Montreal in 1845. In addition to the pie recipe, Mrs. Nourse included several other recipes for gooseberries, including a variety of gooseberry tarts, two different gooseberry fools, preserved gooseberries, and gooseberry wine. Gooseberry fool was a popular light fruity dessert made with cooked, sweetened gooseberries strained through a fine sieve, chilled, and folded together with heavy cream, preferably whipped.

TOAD IN THE HOLE

1 lb. sausages	½ oz. butter
4 oz. flour	pepper & salt
2 eggs	½ pint milk

Grease a small pudding dish with the butter. Prick the sausages and lay them in a dish. Put in the oven for ten minutes. Place the flour in a bowl with pepper & salt, drop into the centre the yolks of eggs. Over this a little milk, stir in the flour from the sides—add the rest of the milk and beat well together. Whip to a stiff froth the whites, the stiffer the better, and add to the batter. When the sausages have been cooked 10 minutes, pour the mixture over and cook ½ hour.

GOOSEBERRY PIE

Pick the gooseberries, fill the dish, and put plenty of sugar over it; cover with a puff paste.

CHAPTER TEN

A Wedding, a Premier, and a Funeral

1851–57

Like the boy who cried wolf, Macdonald threatened to quit politics on such a regular basis that his threats ceased to be taken seriously. His ambivalence likely stemmed from being pulled in many directions and his frustration about being an opposition member while watching his own party, the Conservatives, self-destruct. He was away from the legislature almost as often as he was there, but while there he continued to lobby for Kingston institutions, most notably Queen's University, Regiopolis College, and the Kingston Hospital.

In 1851 Macdonald was re-elected for the third time, still on the opposition side, but now he was one of four local Conservative members, giving the party something of a regional base. From 1851 to 1854, Macdonald lived in a boarding house in Quebec City while the legislature sat. He was waiting for an opportunity to lead the Conservative Party and for the announcement of an election. During these years his drinking problem became significantly more pronounced.

He returned to Kingston from time to time, where Isabella continued to linger in recovery. No one really expected her to make a full recovery. The bigger news was that John's sister, Margaret Macdonald, had accepted a marriage proposal from Reverend James Williamson, a professor at Queen's University. John A. was notified in a telegram sent by his sister Louisa on

October 12, 1852 that Professor Williamson and Margaret would be married on October 19, a mere week later. Macdonald found their haste to marry unseemly. He wrote immediately to Louisa.

Quebec Oct. 13, 1852

My dear Louisa,

I have received your two letters, and I must apologize for not answering the first sooner.

I had no particular reason for not doing so, except that I was very busy and did not anticipate there was any hurry about it.

Mr. Williamson first told me of it, but I had no intimation from him that there was any intention to hurry the marriage. In fact I learnt nothing from him other than the fact of the engagement, with which I expressed my satisfaction.

I said that I thought a careful person, some respectable widow, more a companion than a mere servant should be engaged to act as a an [sic] *attendant for Mamma. I have no idea of imposing her on Mr. Williamson, and depend upon it, it is better that she should remain in her own house. Margaret won't live far from her and can see her every day.*

I shall strain every nerve to be up on the 19th but I am a member the General Election Committee & have taken an oath to attend regularly. . . .

I wish that Moll [Margaret] *shall have a good kit & I wish you to expend £25, for her in such things as you like. Don't say anything to her about it, but when I go up I will settle the bills. Get the things.*

Give my love to Mamma & take it for yourself. I drop a line to Moll.

Yours affectionately,
John A. Macdonald[26]

John A. did not make it to the wedding. Although Margaret's marriage to Williamson should have alleviated her brother from some financial burden, in fact, within four months the newlyweds were so short of money that they moved into the house with Helen and Louisa.

Meanwhile, George Brown, editor of the *Globe* and head of the liberal-leaning Reform Party, was campaigning vigorously for representation by population. The 1851 census had shown that the population of Canada West was greater than that of Canada East. Brown contended that the existing electoral boundaries gave Canada East an unfair advantage in the electoral polls and that "rep by pop," as it became known, would be a fairer system than representation by area. Brown took advantage of his position with the newspaper to publish volumes on the subject, defining it as the critical political issue of the era and pitting French and English against each other.

John A. believed that rep by pop would serve only to alienate the French. During his years in Montreal he had gained a new respect for the French, and he took a different stance from Brown. "Treat them as a nation and they will act as a free people generally do—generously," Macdonald said. "Call them a faction and they will become factious."[27]

Then, out of the blue, in 1854, after three years of polarized opinions and fighting over rep by pop, John A. was dealt a political windfall. The Liberal premier, Francis Hincks, was caught profiting from insider information to the tune of ten thousand pounds. Macdonald seized the opportunity, saying Hincks and his Cabinet were "all steeped to the lips in corruption; that they have no bond of union but the bond of common plunder."[28] With his government in disarray, Hincks had no choice but to dissolve the House and call a general election. Hincks resigned in September 1854, and Conservative Allan McNab was asked to become premier of the Province of Canada and form a new government. Given that there were no Province of Canada-wide parties, MacNab turned the task of building a coalition over to John A., who pulled together a Cabinet of French Canadians, Liberals, right-wing Tories (like MacNab) and moderate "progressive" Conservatives like John A. himself. That coalition was the forerunner to the Progressive Conservative Party of Canada.

MacNab appointed Macdonald as attorney general for Canada West. Now thirty-nine years old, this was the most powerful position Macdonald had held and one he both loved and for which he was well qualified.

It was an interesting time in the development of the country. The economy was booming and a new post-pioneer era was underway. Business was prospering. Banks were opening. Manufacturing towns were springing to life. Grand public buildings were being built. And railway fever had taken ahold of the nation, infecting everyone and especially Premier MacNab. Thanks in part to the Guarantee Act of 1849 that guaranteed bond returns on all railways over seventy-five miles long, a new railway building boom was taking place. The first railway, a seasonal one known as the Champlain and St. Lawrence Railroad, had opened in 1836 to connect river traffic. The building of the Grand Trunk Railway linking Montreal to Sarnia was in full swing. Branch lines and new railway lines were popping up all over the land. The steam engine was having an impact across the colonies. Unfortunately, the growth of new railways was so extensive that it threatened to bankrupt the government.

It was at this point, in 1855, that George-Étienne Cartier joined the Cabinet. Cartier was a fascinating character—handsome, French, and full of himself. He flirted openly and though married, preferred the company of his mistress, who smoked cheroots and wore trousers. Macdonald and Cartier did not immediately see eye to eye. Eventually, united by many factors, including very close political views, Macdonald and Cartier became not just firm friends and allies, but co-leaders of the Conservative Party (1855-73) and the most successful political duo in the history of Canada.

A year after Cartier joined the Cabinet, Allan MacNab, whose popularity had plummeted, was deposed as premier and forced from the Cabinet. This left Macdonald as next in line for the premiership. He assumed this position on November 26, 1857, with George-Étienne Cartier at his side.

Meanwhile John A. had hired a bright new attorney, Archibald Macdonnell, to become a partner in his law firm. Fortunately, Macdonnell was wealthy enough to be able to loan his business partner money to cover some of the company's debts, effectively making Macdonald a debtor to his own employee.

On the home front, Isabella had made a brief attempt to live with John A. in Toronto, in 1855, but illness forced her back to Kingston, into the care of her two servants. She was not well enough to look after little Hugh John so the boy was shuffled between his mother's house on Brock Street and his grandmother's house on Barrie Street, where his aunts Louisa and Margaret lived with his uncle, James Williamson, who was quickly becoming a surrogate father.

Sadly, on December 28, 1857, one month after John A. had been appointed premier of the Province of Canada, Isabella died, bringing to a close a forlorn and unhappy period. John A. and Isabella's marriage had lasted fourteen years and produced two sons. For almost all of those years, Isabella had been ill, an invalid and an opium addict. The obituary in the *Kingston Daily News* was brief.

Funerals in the 1800s were important events. Female family members would be called upon to wash, prepare, and dress the body and lay it in the coffin, which was generally delivered to the home by a local cabinet maker. In this case, Isabella's sister Maria prepared the body for viewing. Family

DIED,

On Monday, the 28th instant, Isabella, wife of the Honorable John A. Macdonald, in the 46th year of her age.

Friends and acquaintances are requested to attend the funeral (without further notice)from his mother's residence, Johnson street, to the Cemetery, on Wednesday, the 30th instant, at one o'clock.

Newspaper Notice of Isabella's Death and Funeral

members hung black crepe across the front door and often over any mirrors as well. Isabella was laid out in the parlour for the invited viewers. It was a tradition for family members and friends to bring food to the grieving family.

Isabella was buried at the Cataraqui Cemetery in Kingston. Later John A. had the coffins of his father, Hugh, and his son John Alexander brought to be with Isabella. Six days after her death, John A. bade farewell to his son Hugh John, leaving him in the care of Margaret and James Williamson.

THE RULES OF MOURNING IN THE 1800s

Most of mourning rules applied to women only. For eighteen months after the funeral, widows were expected to wear a drab black dress, as opposed to a lively or attractive blue-black. They also wore long black veils made of crepe. Men, on the other hand, were expected to wear a black suit for a reasonable period of time and to desist from wearing shiny buttons.

Drinking was paramount. At the funeral, while women rushed around in their black dresses making food, men imbibed, breaking only to eat. Ironically, the food was quite festive. It would not be uncommon to have a couple of roast fowl, a large ham, cooked vegetables, and platters of pickles. There would be fruit pies and puddings and biscuits, and plenty of homemade bread along with butter and cheese. Funerals were occasions for families and the community to eat well and to drink.

Respectable ladies did not generally consume alcohol in public. However, certain occasions merited a little drink, and funeral visitations, because they were held in private homes, were one such occasion. Because Isabella died in winter, it is highly likely that a kettle of mulled wine would have been available at Helen Shaw Macdonald's house. The mulled wine would be drunk from china tea cups to add some respectability. Port and madeira were popular, especially among the British settlers. It is likely that a red wine, such as claret, would have been used. Wine was surprisingly plentiful in the 1800s, and even those on the land had a wide variety of homemade wines utilizing everything from dandelions and nettles to raspberries, damsons, parsnips, and choke cherries.

Here, from *The Cook Not Mad*, is an early recipe for Mulled Wine.

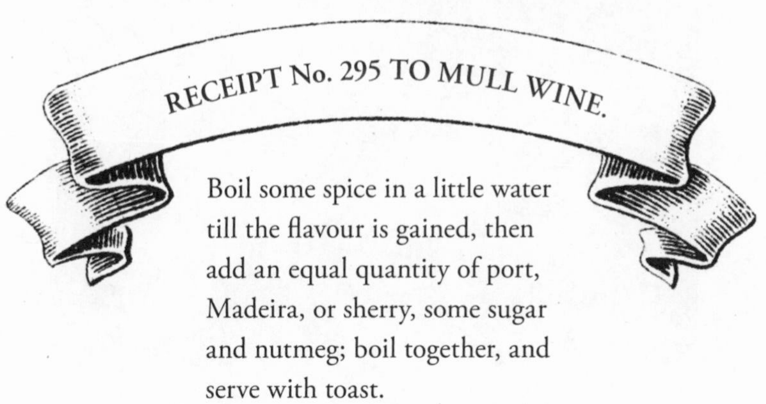

Boil some spice in a little water till the flavour is gained, then add an equal quantity of port, Madeira, or sherry, some sugar and nutmeg; boil together, and serve with toast.

Queen Victoria by Alexander Bassano, 1887.

CHAPTER ELEVEN

We Are Not Amused

1858

Exactly as John A. had predicted, the solution of alternating the capital between Quebec City and Toronto was no solution at all to the question of where the colony's seat of government should reside. Moving the capital every four years—which meant moving all the employees and their families, and all the government paperwork—was impractical, unsettling, costly, and disruptive. Nobody was happy about the situation and a solution seemed nowhere in sight. Placing the capital in either Canada East (Quebec) or Canada West (Ontario) would provoke a furor.

Macdonald put the question to Queen Victoria, asking her to delay her response by several months in the hope that, given some time, the issue might become less contentious. In January 1858, word arrived that Queen Victoria had chosen Ottawa, known previously as Bytown. Some people suggested that the Queen had simply thrown a dart at the map, and Ottawa was where it landed. The truth was that she sought the advice of Governor General Edmund Head, who was, in fact, a Toronto neighbour and close friend of John A. There's no doubt that Ottawa was John A.'s preference.

The monarch's choice, though prudent, made few people happy: Canada East viewed the choice as an English victory; Canada West viewed Ottawa as a sub-arctic backwater, entirely lacking in infrastructure. Macdonald, however, viewed the decision as necessary and less objectionable than any other choice. It was an opportunity for a new start, and it was less offensive than either Toronto or Kingston for Canada East and, likewise, more palatable than either Montreal or Quebec City for Canada West. It was an expedient, though unpopular, choice.

On July 28, 1858, the Assembly debated a response to Queen Victoria's selection that led to one of John A. Macdonald's most famous political manoeuvres—the so-called double shuffle, an incredibly deft and wily piece of political and legal footwork that took a mere four days to complete. It began when George Brown, leader of the opposition, passed a motion that expressed reservations about the suitability of Ottawa as a choice for the capital. Macdonald and his ministers promptly resigned in protest and in deference to the Queen. On July 29, 1858, without the premier and Cabinet, the government fell. The governor general then approached Brown to form the government. Two days later, Brown was ousted and Macdonald was back in power.

The rules of the day stipulated that incoming ministers must resign and subject themselves to by-elections. With the opposition ministers temporarily absent, Brown did not have enough members for a majority in the House. Brown had no choice but to ask Governor General Head for dissolution so an election could be called. Citing prerogative, Head refused and asked Macdonald to re-form the government. Everyone assumed that Macdonald would suffer the identical fate as Brown and that the Government would be again defeated and a general election would have to be called. However, Macdonald knew that there was a parliamentary loophole stipulating that if a minister resigned a Cabinet position and took up a new one within a month, the minister was not required to seek re-election. The rule was designed so that every Cabinet shuffle did not require a costly election. Nobody had ever used it for any other purpose.

Macdonald quickly formed the government, swearing in his old ministers to new Cabinet positions in accordance with the loophole. Since they officially had entirely different portfolios, including Macdonald himself, who was temporarily the postmaster general, they were all exempt from having to resign their seats and run for re-election. The very next day Macdonald shuffled his Cabinet again, moving all the ministers back to their original portfolios, hence the term the *double shuffle.*

The double shuffle proved Macdonald's political sure-footedness and know-how. He was difficult to outsmart even in the most challenging circumstances. Brown, who had goaded him for years, both through his newspaper and in the House, had been served a substantial taste of humble pie. Canada had a new permanent capital. Queen Victoria was smiling. Macdonald had taken another leap up the political ladder.

Macdonald's victory aside, he was still grieving the loss of Isabella. He was lonely and unhappy and drinking to compensate. And as for George Brown, he quit politics and took to a full-time career of raging against Macdonald in the *Globe.* Neither Macdonald nor Brown, it seemed, had much to be amused about.

A QUEEN VICTORIA SANDWICH

Often portrayed as a grim and forbidding character, Victoria was Queen of the United Kingdom of Great Britain from 1837 to 1901. Victoria was also Queen of all the colonies in the British Empire. The young Victoria grew up knowing a lot about Canada as her father, the Duke of Kent, had lived for a decade in Quebec and in Nova Scotia and travelled as far west as Niagara (then Newark).

Eighteen-year-old Victoria ascended to the throne in the same year as the rebellions in Upper and Lower Canada. At her coronation in 1838, an amnesty was granted to the rebels as part of the celebrations. Queen Victoria asked Lord Durham to become Governor-in-Chief of the Province of Canada and to propose a solution to the conflict behind the rebellions. She believed in

Canada as a unified state, "great and prosperous," and favoured confederation for Canada long before it actually came about.

Victoria reigned during a period of great change across most of the world. This was the end of the Industrial Revolution and the beginning of the technological revolution. It was the era of Charles Darwin and his theory of evolution, of vast changes in communications, including the invention of the telegraph and the popular mass press, of power distribution networks, underground sewers, the building of railways, and colonization. All these things had a lasting impact on human society, creating new knowledge and breaking down old structures and replacing them with new ones.

Queen Victoria took most things in life, including food, extremely seriously. A substantial, robust woman, she was an incredibly purposeful and fast eater, and she often finished her course before the others at the table had even been served. Royal protocol dictates that when the monarch finishes, that course is over, regardless of whether the other diners have even started.

It was said that Queen Victoria could eat a six- or seven-course meal in thirty minutes. Dinners were frequently as many as nine courses with up to thirty separate dishes per course. The Queen washed all this down with her favourite drink, a lethally strong mixture of claret and single malt whisky.

On a three-day visit to Hatfield House, a grand country estate in Hertfordshire, England, £70,000 was spent on food and drink for Queen Victoria and her entourage, including £800 worth of turtles for turtle soup and untold thousands of pounds for the finest champagne, wine, and whisky. Queen Victoria and John A. shared a similar love of fine food and alcohol. Victoria had many peccadillos, among them an insistence on eating with all the windows open no matter the season. She also liked silence or, at the very least, a lack of all frivolity at the table. Once when someone dared to tell a funny story at dinner, Queen Victoria put an immediate end to any such folly. "We are not amused," she said, bluntly, silencing everyone immediately. Apparently such foolishness disrupted her concentration and digestion.

The tradition of taking afternoon tea was introduced to Queen Victoria by the Duchess of Bedford. Victoria, who had a hard time lasting from the noon meal until dinner in the evening, found a pot of tea and some light cakes in the late afternoon useful for maintaining her energy. Her favourite cake was a sponge, sandwiched together with jam and thickened cream, and dredged with sugar. This cake has subsequently become known as a Victoria sponge or a Victoria sandwich cake.

The following is Mrs. Beeton's recipe as it appeared in the 1874 version of her cookbook. Mrs. Beeton, who culinary historians say was a better copier and plagiarizer than a cook, apparently accidentally left the eggs out of her 1861 version, calling even her copying skills into question.

In later versions of her book, Mrs. Beeton's recipe for Victoria sandwiches continued to evolve. By 1912 she had scaled back the amount of butter and sugar and added milk and baking powder. The version included here is interesting because it is a handy scalable formula according to the number and weight of eggs, which dictates the amount of butter, sugar, and flour required, making it easy to reduce or increase the recipe as desired. The recipe calls for pounded sugar because during the Victorian era sugar was sold in loaves which had to be made into powder for use in recipes or cut into cubes for tea and coffee.

Isabella Beeton's books sold an astonishing number of copies. It probably didn't hurt that she had married wealthy publisher Samuel Beeton when she was just twenty years old. The first version of her book sold over sixty thousand copies in its first year of publication and nearly two million copies by 1868. Even by modern standards, those numbers are impressive. *Mrs. Beeton's Book of House Management* remains one of the most successful cookbooks of all time and a definitive source of information about food and culinary history in the nineteenth and twentieth centuries.

VICTORIA SANDWICHES.

Ingredients.—4 eggs; their weight in pounded sugar, butter and flour; 1/4 spoonful of salt, a layer of any kind of jam or marmalade.

Mode.—Beat the butter to a cream; dredge in the flour and pounded sugar; stir these ingredients well together, and add the eggs, which should be previously thoroughly whisked. When the mixture has been well beaten for about 10 minutes, butter a Yorkshire-pudding tin, pour in the batter, and bake it in a moderate oven for 20 minutes. Let it cool, spread one half of the cake with a layer of nice preserve, place over it the other half of the cake, press the pieces slightly together, and then cut it into long finger-pieces; pile them in cross bars on a glass dish, and serve.

Time.—20 minutes. Average cost, 1s 3d

Sufficient for 5 or 6 persons.

Seasonable at any time.

CHAPTER TWELVE

The Born-Again Bachelor

1858–60

There were many reasons why 1858 was an arduous year for John A. He was mourning the death of Isabella in late 1857, and his mother was still in very poor health. Following the double shuffle, the sessions in Parliament were some of the nastiest and most vitriolic on record. As an escape, Macdonald took to going on drunken benders that lasted for days. While his drinking problem was neither new nor secret, it was becomingly increasingly problematic. With Isabella gone, he scarcely bothered to return home to Kingston; instead, he would send letters to his sisters with instructions for Hugh John's care, and he spent weekends drinking himself into a stupor.

Macdonald's letters home spoke volumes about his state of mind. In March 1858, he wrote,

> *My dear Margaret,*
>
> *I was very unwell last week so as to be confined to bed for three days and was hardly able to crawl to the House, when it opened....*
>
> *We are having a hard fight in the House & will beat them in the votes, but it will, I think end in my retiring as soon as I can*

with honour. I find the work & annoyance too much for me...
Affectionately yours
John A. Macdonald

Love to the parson.[29]

In May 1858, Macdonald delivered a rambling, incoherent, and very likely drunken speech in the Legislature. Afterwards he admitted that he was "not altogether free of blame," and joined the Temperance Society, thereby provoking a round of scathing mockery from the *Globe*. Not surprisingly, his fling with the Temperance Society didn't amount to much. Macdonald was a binge drinker, and a very open one at that. At a public meeting where he was heckled for being intoxicated, he famously quipped, "Yes, but the people prefer John A. drunk to George Brown sober." There was an element of truth to this.

In the summer of 1859, John A. was aboard the steamboat *Ploughboy* heading from Collingwood to Sault St. Marie when the ship's engine failed and the vessel had to cut off its steam. For the better part of two days, the boat pitched and tossed in gale force winds, eventually travelling perilously close to the dramatic rocky coast of Cabot Head on the Bruce Peninsula. The crew threw out anchors hoping to prevent the boat from running into the rocks, but the anchors were futile in the deep waters of Georgian Bay. Finally, about forty metres from shore, in water fifty-five metres deep, an anchor caught the bottom and the boat and its passengers were saved from disaster. John A. wrote to his sister:

Toronto July 7, 1859

My dear Margaret,

You will see by the papers what a narrow escape we had. None of the party will again be nearer their graves until they are placed in them. The people behaved well, the women heroically.

I am none the worse for the trip. The Governor General will be here tonight and I hope then [to be] *free in a few days to get away to Kingston.*

Love to Mamma, Hughy and Loo not forgetting the Parson.

Yours always,
John A.[30]

Clearly the trip had shaken him. If nothing else he must have realized that when he died, Hugh John would be an orphan, and so in short order he made out his will. In a letter to Louisa, he laid out his wishes, stating that no decision was to be made until their mother's death and then at that time, both Louisa and Margaret would receive seventy-five pounds annually, as well as an allowance for "Hughey."

The terms were not especially generous, but then Macdonald's financial situation was precarious. In August 1859, one of his properties was seized for auction in order to pay off some debts. There were those who wondered how such an intelligent man could be so reckless with money. A Kingston real estate development partner said, "Macdonald has all but ruined me by his wretched carelessness."[31]

By late 1859, an appropriate amount of time since Isabella's death, Macdonald had begun publicly to express an interest in having a relationship with a woman. He set about organizing a Valentine's Day Ball for February 14, 1860, to be held in the grand music hall of the St. Louis Hotel in Quebec

City. He invited a thousand guests to pay one dollar apiece to attend; however, none of his family members made it to the event. The expense and the time involved were too much for them, given that they were looking after the ailing Helen Macdonald and young Hugh. The family were watching every penny while John A. was, as always, spending faster than his income allowed.

Macdonald organized for the elegant mirror-lined music hall to be filled with garlands of roses and wreaths of flowers, along with busts of Queen Victoria and the Prince of Wales. Gas-lit chandeliers glowed as a fountain sprayed guests with eau de cologne. Eight hundred attendees were treated to liberal quantities of champagne, sparkling wine, sherry, port, and ale. Every woman at the party received a handwritten valentine from Macdonald. At dinner a huge pie was wheeled into the ballroom, and as the orchestra played, twenty-four live blackbirds were released from the pie. The drinking and socializing and dancing went on into well into the night, and no expense was spared.

Macdonald loved a good party and a bit of frivolity from time to time. It's possible that this event was planned by Macdonald to impress the world at large or some woman in particular. Possibly he was seeking a new wife. There were rumours of women in his life, in particular, Susan Agnes Bernard, and also Elizabeth Hall, a widow whose late husband's legal affairs had been settled by John A. in 1858. In December 1860, Elizabeth wrote a gushing and flirtatious letter to John A. which began with the phrase, "My beloved John," and ended with, "Goodbye my own darling—love from loving Lizzie."[32] She could not have imagined at the time that her correspondence would become part of the national archives.

Macdonald had always been popular with women. At forty-five he had grown into his unusual looks. With his cravats and long, wild hair and prominent nose, he was certainly striking, but it was undoubtedly his wit, intelligence, gregariousness, and, now more than ever, his political position that were so alluring.

The next significant public event for Macdonald was the Prince of Wales's tour in 1860, bringing Queen Victoria's eighteen-year-old son, Albert Edward, on his first royal tour of the colony. John A. met the prince's boat in Gaspé on August 10, and in the weeks to follow, he toured with Prince Albert through Quebec City, Montreal, Arnprior, Almonte, and Brockville before finally heading to Kingston. The tour was a grand triumph with Canada sparkling in the summer sun. There were official bridge openings and enthusiastic, welcoming crowds and lavish champagne receptions and dinners. Everything went off without a hitch until the royal steamboat with its entourage reached Kingston, where Macdonald had planned a grand ball in honour of the prince. There on the Kingston shoreline were fifteen thousand Orangemen assembled en masse in costumes, along with signs and a banner, to meet the prince. This was an unexpected and unwelcome event on a scale that could not be ignored. It was symptomatic of the tensions between Roman Catholic Lower Canada (Quebec) and the Protestant population of Upper Canada. John A. insisted that the Loyal Orange Order was perfectly legal in Canada and that the prince had been welcomed in French in Quebec and had toured Roman Catholic institutions while there. It was a valid point but the prince was not having any of it. The prince never disembarked from the boat. The Loyal Orange Order was illegal in Britain, and Prince Albert was not about to break the laws of his own country by greeting them on what he thought of as British soil. The royal party stayed aboard the boat, and the Orangemen refused to leave the shore. Thus, after a twenty-four hour standoff, the ship sailed off to Belleville to the prince's next event. Macdonald's royal gala dinner was a complete and very awkward bust. For the next two weeks, he snubbed the royal tour and was presumed to be on a drinking binge somewhere. In due course the prince travelled to the United States, where he finished off his tour before returning to Britain.

The *Globe* accused Macdonald of incompetence. Macdonald retaliated by heading off on an extended speaking tour throughout Canada West in an attempt to win back the voters by establishing himself as a man of the people. The trip was a huge success. Macdonald was warm and engaging—more a storyteller than an orator. He was a natural with an audience, inviting participation and answering questions honestly. He met people in towns and villages and rural settings. There were many lunches and dinners, often with several courses. Macdonald used these occasions to talk to as many people as he could. He attended picnics and visited farms. And everywhere he went he left his audiences charmed.

One of the highlights of the tour was when he climbed atop a piece of farm machinery to give his address, and when advised that he was standing on a manure spreader, Macdonald beamed at the audience and said, "This is the first time I've stood on a Liberal platform." The crowd loved him. George Brown's scathing attacks could never compete.

STUMP SPEECHES AND COMMUNITY PICNICS

John A. Macdonald was the first Canadian politician to take his political message on the road. The custom began in the United States, where political candidates travelled between towns campaigning and delivering their addresses, often using a tree stump as a speaking platform, resulting in the term *stump speech*.

Macdonald was exceptionally good at getting his message across with a mixture of information, familiarity, and humour. Since mass communication was limited to newspapers and there was little else in the way of entertainment, villagers and farmers alike turned out in great numbers to hear what he had to say. The crowds stayed on for the dinners and picnics.

Picnics were celebratory events in the Victorian era, and they often lasted all day and well into the evening. Great effort went into the preparation. In an era where taking a vacation was almost unheard of for most families,

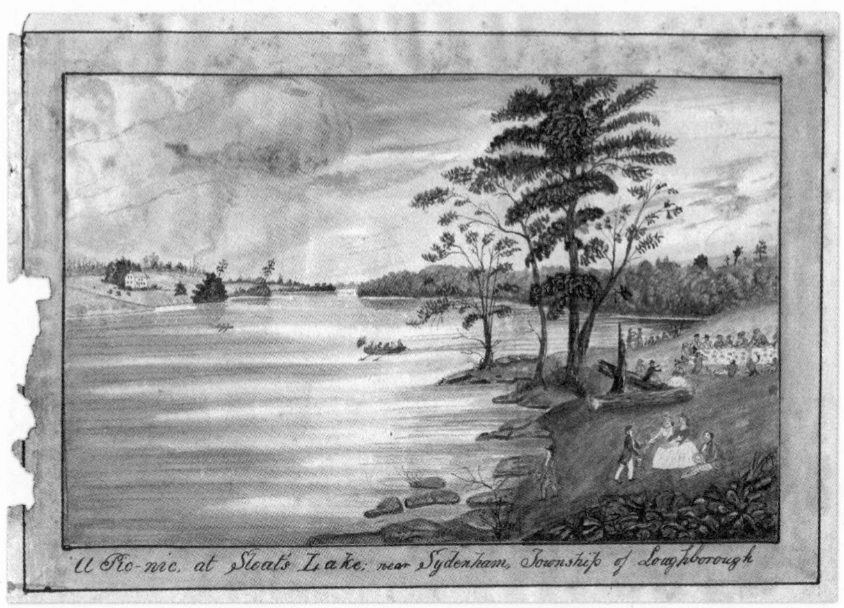

A Pic-nic, at Sloat's Lake; near Sydenham, Township of Loughborough, 1861
by Thomas Burrowes

picnics were valuable opportunities for young and old to meet to share food and news and take a much-needed break from chores and work.

The following comprehensive instructions for a Victorian picnic come directly from Mrs. Beeton's 1861 book. Note the vast quantity of alcohol specified for forty people.

BILL OF FARE FOR A PICNIC FOR 40 PERSONS.

A joint of cold roast beef, a joint of cold boiled beef, 2 ribs of lamb, 2 shoulders of lamb, 4 roast fowls, 2 roast ducks, 1 ham, 1 tongue, 2 veal-and-ham pies, 2 pigeon pies, 6 medium-sized lobsters, 1 piece of collared calf's head, 18 lettuces, 6 baskets of salad, 6 cucumbers.

Stewed fruit well sweetened, and put into glass bottles well corked; 3 or 4 dozen plain pastry biscuits to eat with the stewed fruit, 2 dozen fruit turnovers, 4 dozen cheesecakes, 2 cold cabinet puddings in moulds, 2 blancmanges in moulds, a few jam puffs, 1 large cold plum-pudding (this must be good), a few baskets of fresh fruit, 3 dozen plain biscuits, a piece of cheese, 6 lbs. of butter (this, of course, includes the butter for tea), 4 quarter loaves of household bread, 3 dozen rolls, 6 loaves of tin bread (for tea), 2 plain plum cakes, 2 pound cakes, 2 sponge cakes, a tin of mixed biscuits, 1/2 lb, of tea. Coffee is not suitable for a picnic, being difficult to make.

THINGS NOT TO BE FORGOTTEN AT A PICNIC.

A stick of horseradish, a bottle of mint-sauce well corked, a bottle of salad dressing, a bottle of vinegar, made mustard, pepper, salt, good oil, and pounded sugar. If it can be managed, take a little ice. It is scarcely necessary to say that plates, tumblers, wine-glasses, knives, forks, and spoons, must not be forgotten; as also teacups and saucers, 3 or 4 teapots, some lump sugar, and milk, if this last-named article cannot be obtained in the neighbourhood. Take 3 corkscrews.

Beverages: 3 dozen quart bottles of ale, packed in hampers; ginger-beer, soda-water, and lemonade, of each 2 dozen bottles; 6 bottles of sherry, 6 bottles of claret, champagne at discretion, and any other light wine that may be preferred, and 2 bottles of brandy. Water can usually be obtained so it is useless to take it.

CHAPTER THIRTEEN

The Birth of Confederation

1861–64

In the 1861 general election, John A. found himself in a tight battle for his seat, running against his former schoolmate Oliver Mowat. The fight was nasty, with raised fists and blows and slurs between the two sides. In a moment of ill temper after an accusation by Mowat in the assembly, Macdonald rose from his seat and roared across the floor shouting, "You damn pup! I'll slap your chops."[33] Mowat, a plump, bespectacled, teetotalling do-gooder had pushed his former childhood friend too far.

At one point, Mowat's supporters attacked a school where John A. was speaking, hurling rocks at the windows. Inside, the audience took shelter, but the damage was done. Macdonald's authority was undermined, his speech was ruined, and any semblance of friendship with Mowat was shattered, along with the glass in the schoolhouse windows.

The real battle of the election was the old issue of rep by pop. John A. clung stubbornly to his stance that this would not serve the interests of the union because it alienated Canada East, which had the smaller population. Mowat was on the other side—vociferously arguing in favour of rep by pop.

In the end, Macdonald held his seat by a much slimmer margin than he was used to. When the votes were tallied, three days after the election, John A. had 758 votes and Mowat had 474. He celebrated his victory at Hazeldell, the home in Portsmouth Village, where his mother and family were living. He arrived in a beautifully decorated carriage drawn by six horses followed by a procession of over a hundred carriages. Eighty-four-year-old Helen Macdonald helped prepare the victory meal — "a bountiful collation was spread on tables beneath the pleasant shade of the trees,"[34] — the last one she would ever celebrate.

On the plus side, Macdonald had just won his first Conservative majority government, and as an added bonus, George Brown, who had re-entered the political arena, had lost Toronto. Nevertheless, the victory also came at a high personal price. Severely criticized about his alcohol consumption, Macdonald once again joined the Temperance Society.

By November 1861, with the American Civil War in full swing, Britain had become nervous about Canada's vulnerability. There was good reason for fear. Many Americans, including Thomas Jefferson, a founding father of the United States and the third president, had been open about the possibility of "annexation to liberate Canada." Macdonald was adamant this would never happen, swearing his allegiance to a unified Canada and Britain.

Irish-born journalist Thomas D'Arcy McGee, who had lived in the United States before moving to Canada, was in agreement with Macdonald. "They coveted Florida, and seized it; they coveted Louisiana, and purchased it; and they picked a quarrel with Mexico, which ended by their getting California," said McGee. "They sometimes pretended to despise these [British North American] colonies as prizes beneath their ambition; but had we not the strong arm of England over us, we should not have had a separate existence."[35]

With tensions rising and the possibility that if the North won the American Civil War, an invasion into Canada might follow, England asked Canada to make some contributions to its own defence capabilities. In response, Macdonald tabled the Militia Bill, an ambiguous piece of legislation that would cost the equivalent of one tenth of government revenues. On May 20, 1862, the bill was defeated by sixty-one to fifty-four. The following day, Macdonald and Cartier both stepped down, and Liberal leader John Sandfield Macdonald was appointed the new premier.

John A. had been absent for much of the debate about the bill. It turned out that he had been on an extended drinking session. The *Globe* stepped up its attacks, no longer describing a very drunk Macdonald as being "in a state of wild excitement" but now using the phrase that John A. Macdonald was having "one of his old attacks." Even Lord Monck, the governor general, weighed in on the subject, saying that Macdonald's absences were caused "nominally by illness, but really, as everyone knows, by drunkenness."[36] Macdonald feigned cheerful indifference, claiming he was glad of a respite and calling his defeat "a grateful tonic." He wrote to his sister to explain himself.

Quebec, May 23, 1862

My dear Margaret,

You complain of my not having written. It is true but I had the excuse of overwork. I no longer have that. You will have seen that I am out of office. I am at last free thank God!...

If I had chosen this mode of falling; I would have selected the way in which we were defeated....

I have been very ill but am crawling around....You must have my room ready. I don't know when I may be up to take possession.

Give my love to the whole house hold & believe me my dear Magt,

Yours affectionately,
J.A. MD.[37]

Not long after this, John A. arrived back in Kingston, hoping to earn some money working in his law office. Less than five months later, on October 24, 1862, Helen Macdonald died. Immediately following her funeral, Macdonald set off once again for England, where he stayed until February 1863. He was biding his time. But he also had another mission—he wanted to know where he stood with British officials. Amazingly, despite the fact that news of his drinking problem had reached Britain, he was feted everywhere he went and asked if he would consider leading the Conservatives again.

Macdonald didn't have to wait long. In May 1863, Premier Sandfield Macdonald's Liberal government was dissolved, and after a series of parliamentary deadlocks and through some fancy political wrangling, by December, John A. Macdonald found himself re-elected. He had banded with former Liberal turned Conservative D'Arcy McGee. The pair, one as bad as the other, campaigned by day and ate and drank all night long. Their nights generally culminated in rowdy sing-songs, a favourite of which went along these lines: "A drunken man is a terrible curse, But a drunken woman is twice as worse."[38]

By March 30, 1864, a Conservative government was in power with Etienne Taché as the titular leader. Behind him, Macdonald and Cartier were back in business, but not for long. Ten weeks later, on June 14, the Conservatives were defeated in the House. Deadlock was complete once again, in a similar set of circumstances to those that preceded both the 1858 double shuffle and the dissolution of Premier Sandfield's government of 1863.

Between 1854 and 1864, deadlock had become a major problem for the government because of the so-called double majority requirement established under the 1840 Act of Union, which specified that in order for a bill to pass in the Legislative Assembly, there had to be a vote in both Canada East and Canada West. Since the two sides could rarely agree, votes frequently ended in stalemates, referred to as deadlock.

In addition, the government was technically bankrupt. Lurching from deadlock to deadlock and the subsequent changes of governments that ensued was a costly and ineffective way to run a country and proof that the government of the Province of Canada was, at least in its present form, unworkable.

Despite his foibles, all eyes turned towards John A. Macdonald because he had enough political acumen to create a government that could operate for both Canada East and West. Nevertheless, the solution came from George Brown, who had risen up from the ashes yet again, and proposed a Great Coalition government that would work towards a confederation of all the regions of British North America from the Maritimes to the North-West to Upper and Lower Canada. Macdonald, who had previously supported coalition of Canada East and West rather than a confederation, was forced to agree with his old rival. Besides, his love of power helped convince him to promote the idea of a confederation and thus maintain his political career.

The Taché-Macdonald-Cartier government joined with Brown, McGee, and Alexander Galt, making John A. as the principal architect of the proposed confederation. In August 1864, the Canadian government steamer *Queen Victoria*, loaded to the gunnels with champagne, sailed into Charlottetown, Prince Edward Island for the Charlottetown Conference, an event that became a turning point in the history of Canada.

The conference was attended by representatives from Canada East and Canada West, New Brunswick, Nova Scotia, and Prince Edward Island. Incredibly, each of the five colonies had its own Legislative Assembly, elected officials, lieutenant-governor, coinage, stamps, and customs duties. Macdonald, Cartier, Brown, and Galt took turns outlining their ideas for confederation. Cartier and Macdonald both made major speeches about the virtues of confederation and the different types of federal governments.

Banquets, lunches, dinners, and late-night drinking sessions paved the way to new allegiances, although old rivalries lurked in the background. Macdonald was said to be "crotchety": he arrived for a Cabinet meeting "half drunk" and when more ale arrived, he apparently became cantankerous. The meeting broke up when Macdonald and Brown began to argue about contracts for the new Parliament buildings in Ottawa.[39] The Charlottetown

Islander recorded a buffet dinner that included "substantials of beef rounds, splendid hams, salmon, lobster... all vegetable delicacies... pastry in all its forms, fruits in almost every variety."[40]

The conference moved from Prince Edward Island to Halifax, then to Saint John, and finally to Fredericton. More champagne and more banquets ensued. The glittering concept of a united Canada was fast taking hold and so, on October 10, 1864, a second conference, the Quebec Conference, was held in Quebec City. During the two weeks that followed, Macdonald rallied the separate parties with impassioned speeches. His appeal was directed not only to Canadians but also to England and the United States. American power was a reality that had to be contended with. Only a united Canada would have the power to withstand it.

"For the sake of securing peace to ourselves and our posterity," he said, "We must make ourselves powerful. The great security for peace is to convince the world of our strength by being united."[41]

There were the usual hiccups. It was at the Quebec Conference that Frances Monck, the governor general's niece, noted that Macdonald was always drunk and that he had been found in his hotel room, with a rug thrown over his nightshirt, practising Hamlet in a looking glass.[42] Nonetheless, while he wasn't drinking and playing at being Hamlet, Macdonald was remarkably productive. In two weeks he drafted resolutions from the concepts raised at Charlottetown. These seventy-two resolutions outlined the division of powers and responsibilities between the provinces and the federal government. Cartier wanted to see provincial powers and rights to guarantee that each province could retain its own distinctness. Macdonald on the other hand advocated for a strong, central federal government. The balance they arrived at is still largely in place today. The resolutions also outlined how Parliament would work, with an elected House of Commons based on representation by population and an appointed Senate. By October 27, 1864, amidst much partying, feasting, and drinking, the draft constitution was approved, laying the foundation for the British North America Act and the birth of a new nation.

EARLY RECIPE FOR CONFEDERATION

The basic recipe seemed to be three parts champagne to two parts food to one part everything else, including political discussions, boating, and dancing. The Charlottetown Conference in particular was an anticipatory celebration of what might lie ahead for the new nation. From the time the *Queen Victoria* docked, there was an endless round of talks, drinks, dances, and feasts. Throughout the literature pertaining to the confederation conferences are numerous references to the abundance of food and alcohol. No expense was spared at these most critical of political conferences.

This passage from "The Charlottetown Conference and its Significance in Canadian History," paints a vivid picture of how the delegates were received:

> The Provincial Building, where the Conference had held its sittings, was hurriedly prepared for the festivities during the absence of the delegates. The Legislative Council Chamber was fitted up as a reception room. The legislative library served as refreshment room where copious quantities of tea, coffee, sherry, and champagne were available. The Assembly, where the dancing took place, was gaily decorated with flags, evergreens, and flowers, and with the most brilliant lighting effects that the superintendent of the local gas works, Mr. Murphy, could produce. The early part of the evening was spent dancing. Mrs. Dundas and John A. Macdonald and Lieutenant Governor Dundas and Mrs. T. H. Haviland led off the first quadrille. At one o'clock the party withdrew to the Council Chamber where they found the table "literally

> groaning under the choicest foods," the proposal and response to toasts continued until after three o'clock in the morning. All the delegates then repaired to the Queen Victoria which was to convoy the entire Conference across the straits to Nova Scotia.[43]

Others wrote in a similar vein of twelve-course meals and grand buffets of oysters, lobsters, and other island delicacies, all well lubricated with champagne. Lobster enjoyed a resurgence in popularity in the 1800s after a spate of unpopularity in the 1600s and 1700s, when lobsters were so plentiful that settlers complained of having only lobsters to eat. Oysters, however, were always a prized delicacy, especially by the British, regardless of class. Typically oysters were served cooked, often stewed or fried. This simple, elegant recipe from *The Cook Not Mad* is a near-perfect treatment for freshly shucked oysters. Champagne, of course, is the ideal accompaniment.

No. 27. OYSTERS FRIED

Simmer them in their own liquor for a couple of minutes, take them out and lay them on a cloth to drain, and then flour them, egg and bread crumb them, put them into boiling fat and fry them a delicate brown.

CHAPTER FOURTEEN

Macdonald Is on Fire

1865–66

Early in 1865, Macdonald locked both himself and the boarding-house cat in his room and proceeded to practise his opening speech for the upcoming parliamentary debate on confederation, with the cat as his audience.[44] The most unusual part of all this was that Macdonald rarely, if ever, rehearsed a speech. One of his great skills was his ability to speak off the cuff, without notes.

This speech was apparently one of the longest and least convincing he ever gave. Among other things, Macdonald argued that confederation was an opportunity that might never recur and warned of the danger of impending anarchy. The debate continued until March 11, 1865, when, at 4:30 in the morning, the vote on the seventy-two resolutions was finally called and handily passed. It is possible that success was inevitable because everyone just needed to get to bed after nearly two months of confederation overload. Now it only needed to pass the British Parliament before becoming law.

With the session over, once again Macdonald packed his bags and left for England. He was travelling with a delegation of colleagues, including George-Étienne Cartier, John Alexander Galt, and George Brown. Their mission was to rally imperial support for the new nation. Choosing George Brown to go along was a strategic move on Macdonald's part. It was a way of patching up their badly frayed relationship while simultaneously proving to the British that confederation was a joint decision, stretching across personalities, parties, and provinces.

The delegation was presented to Queen Victoria. They dined night after night in the mansions of dukes and lords and attended Derby Day at Epsom Downs, where even George Brown managed to get into the spirit of things and fire peas from his pea-shooter at the neighbouring open carriages. While they were at the races, the four Canadians, who had taken along a picnic hamper from Fortnum and Mason, hobnobbed with socialites, dined on turtle soup, and drank champagne cup, an elegant champagne cocktail.

Macdonald spent a day at Oxford where he received an honorary doctor of laws degree and promptly wrote to Louisa to brag a little, telling her, "This is the greatest honour they can confer, and is much sought after by the first men."[45]

The delegation arrived home on July 7, 1865, with their mission accomplished, which was easily enough done since their mission had been entirely ambiguous. Three weeks later, Premier Étienne Taché died, and Governor General Monck appointed Macdonald as first minister. Brown balked. He was, he insisted, Macdonald's equal and should have had the same opportunity. Monck promptly ousted Macdonald and appointed Sir Narcisse-Fortunat Belleau, a former member of the Cabinet, as Tache's successor. Poor Brown still wasn't satisfied. He complained that Macdonald and Cartier were slighting him, and he quit speaking to Macdonald.

By December 1865, Brown had had enough. He quit politics again. He headed straight back to Toronto and the *Globe*, where he continued his endless griping about the government, in particular about the drinking habits of John A. Macdonald.

With uncertainty and rancour taking hold of the government once again, the Maritime provinces all but withdrew their intent to join Confederation. However, as sometimes happens, a threat from another quarter had a significant influence on the progress of the creation of a new nation. It came from the Fenians, an organization of Irish nationalists who sought to undermine the British presence in North America. They presented a very real threat to Canada, and not just in the Maritimes.

The first Fenian raid took place at Campobello Island, New Brunswick, in April 1866. Seven hundred-plus Fenians had assembled on the Maine shore across from the island but, due to logistical bumbling, had to wait for their weapons to arrive. Their large numbers alerted authorities and while the Fenians waited, the New Brunswick militia and six Royal Navy warships mustered in the area. When the Fenians finally attacked, they fled after firing only a few shots. No causalities ensued, although a British flag was stolen and a few buildings sustained fire damage.

On June 2, 1866, the Fenians, under Colonel John O'Neill, staged the Battle at Ridgeway (near Niagara Falls) and killed nine Canadians and injured thirty others. The attack was rumoured to be just the beginning, and newspapers warned of much worse to come, with the possibility of as many as 1,500 heavily armed Fenians crossing the Niagara River into Canada.

These initial attacks convinced most Canadians of the value of confederation. Despite the Fenians' failure in the Campobello Island attack, the raid did help swing public opinion in New Brunswick in favour of confederation. In the provincial elections that took place in spring 1866, the anti-confederation government in New Brunswick was defeated and replaced with a pro-confederation one, paving the way for the final step: Britain's approval of the British North America Bill.

A final conference in London was required to work out any remaining details before the matter was voted on in Westminster. On July 19, 1866, the East Coast delegation set sail for London. Meanwhile, Macdonald languished in Ottawa, refusing to budge. He rarely surfaced, though stories circulated that he was spending all his time in Ottawa's Russell House Hotel and was now permanently drunk.[46]

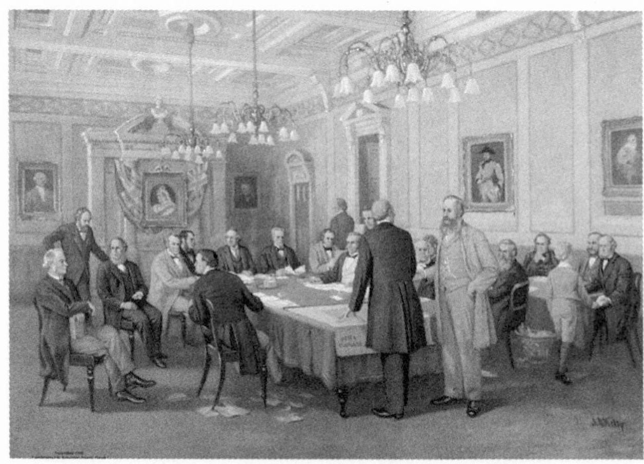

The Fathers of Confederation at the London Conference

In mid-August 1866, the *Globe* launched a public attack, alleging that for three days in a row Macdonald appeared in the House completely and utterly "gone" and unconscious of what he was doing, and further, that Macdonald and a Cabinet colleague (unnamed but thought to be D'Arcy McGee) were seen rolling helplessly on the ministerial benches.

Finally, on November 14, four months after the rest of the delegation, Macdonald managed to pull himself together and set sail for England. His travelling companions included his friend and ally Cartier, Alexander Galt, Hector-Louis Langevin, and two Reform ministers. The final confederation conference began on December 4, 1866 at London's Westminister Palace Hotel and lasted three days. Shortly after the conference ended, the British House of Commons and House of Lords recessed for the Christmas and New Year break, and the Canadian delegation had little choice but to wait in London for Parliament to resume and vote on the British North America Bill.

At Macdonald's recommendation, no minutes were taken at the London

Conference and publicity was avoided. At least, most publicity was avoided. By the end of December, Macdonald had managed to light both himself and his hotel room on fire. He wrote to reassure his sister Louisa.

London, Dec. 27, 1866

My dear Louisa,

... For fear that such an alarming story may reach you, I may as well tell you as it occurred. Cartier, Galt & myself returned from Lord Carnarvon's place in the country late at night. I went to bed but commenced reading the newspapers of the day, after my usual fashion. I fell asleep & was wakened by intense heat. I found my bed, bed clothes & curtains all on fire.

I didn't lose my presence of mind, pulled down the curtains with my hands, and extinguished them with the water in my room. The pillow was burnt under my head and bolster as well. All the bed clothes were blazing. I dragged them all off on the floor & knowing the action of feathers on flame, I ripped open bolster and pillows and poured an avalanche of feather on the blazing mass, & then stamped out the fire with my hands & feet. Lest the mattress might be burning internally I then went to Cartier's bedroom, & with his assistance carried all the water in three adjoining rooms into mine, & finally extinguished all appearance of fire. We made no alarm & only Cartier, Galt & myself knew of the accident. After it was all over, it was then discovered that I had been on fire. My shirt was burnt on my back & my hair, forehead & hands scorched. Had I not worn a very thick flannel shirt under my nightshirt, I would have been burnt to death, as it was my escape was miraculous.

. . . I had a merry Xmas alone in my own room and my dinner of tea & toast & drank to all your healths in bohea, though you didn't deserve it.

. . . Love to Hugh, Magt & the Parson & believe me,

Affectionately yours,
John A. Macdonald[47]

THE VICTORIAN PROCLIVITY FOR ALCOHOL

Despite the depictions of the Victorian era as morally upright and sexually repressed, the use of alcohol and drugs was so prevalent that it might be described as rampant. Even Queen Victoria's servants were allocated eight pints of beer a day—though they were required to drink it "below stairs." Granted, beer was slightly lower in alcohol than it is today but the eight pints were only the allocated ration. Many began drinking at breakfast. Beer and other forms of alcohol were generally regarded as safer than water because they were less likely to carry dangerous pathogens.

Public drunkenness in both Great Britain and in the colonies was common, especially amongst the working class, which generally consumed beer, cider, and gin. The middle and upper classes drank wine, scotch, and brandy. The irony was that drunkenness was likely as prevalent in the upper classes, however they were less apt to be found in public, in part because their houses afforded them privacy.

When the Temperance Society began stepping up its campaign against the consumption of alcohol Queen Victoria was said to have been outraged. In his book *Everyday Drinking: The Distilled Kingsley Amis,* Amis writes, "the Great Queen was 'violently opposed to teetotalism, consenting to have one cleric promoted to a deanery only if he promised to stop advocating the pernicious heresy.'"

John A. was known to drink the occasional ale, glass of brandy, or tumbler full of gin, which could be handily disguised as a glass of water, but his favourite tipple was wine, usually claret (also known as Bordeaux) or champagne. His fondness for champagne was a fashionable choice. By the mid-1800s it was tremendously popular among the upper classes in Britain and the colonies. England's growing taste for wine was fed by the French wine industry, which helped usher in a productive period in this cornerstone of the French economy.

Champagne cup was a cocktail that was deemed suitable for celebratory occasions. In the first edition of her book, Mrs. Beeton included the following recipe and notes about champagne. In subsequent editions, she included a wide variety of cup renditions, including recipes for a badminton cup, claret cup, and a Parisian champagne cup.

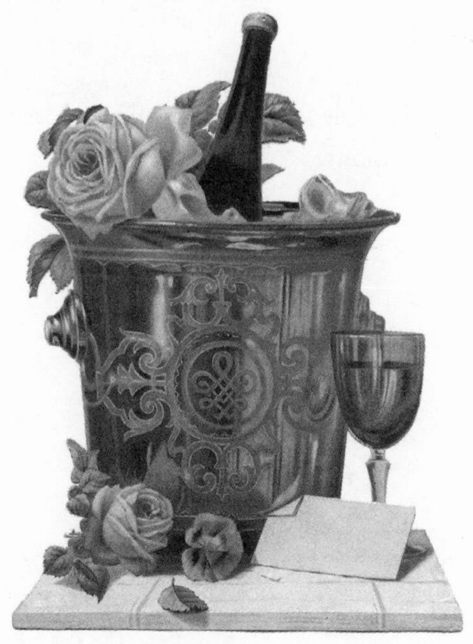

CHAMPAGNE-CUP

1832. INGREDIENTS.—1 quart bottle of champagne, 2 bottles of soda-water, 1 liqueur-glass of brandy or Curaçoa, 2 tablespoonfuls of powdered sugar, 1 lb. of pounded ice, a sprig of green borage.

Mode.—Put all the ingredients into a silver cup; stir them together, and serve the same as claret-cup No. 1831. Should the above proportion of sugar not be found sufficient to suit some tastes, increase the quantity. When borage is not easily obtainable, substitute for it a few slices of cucumber-rind.

Seasonable.—Suitable for pic-nics, balls, weddings, and other festive occasions.

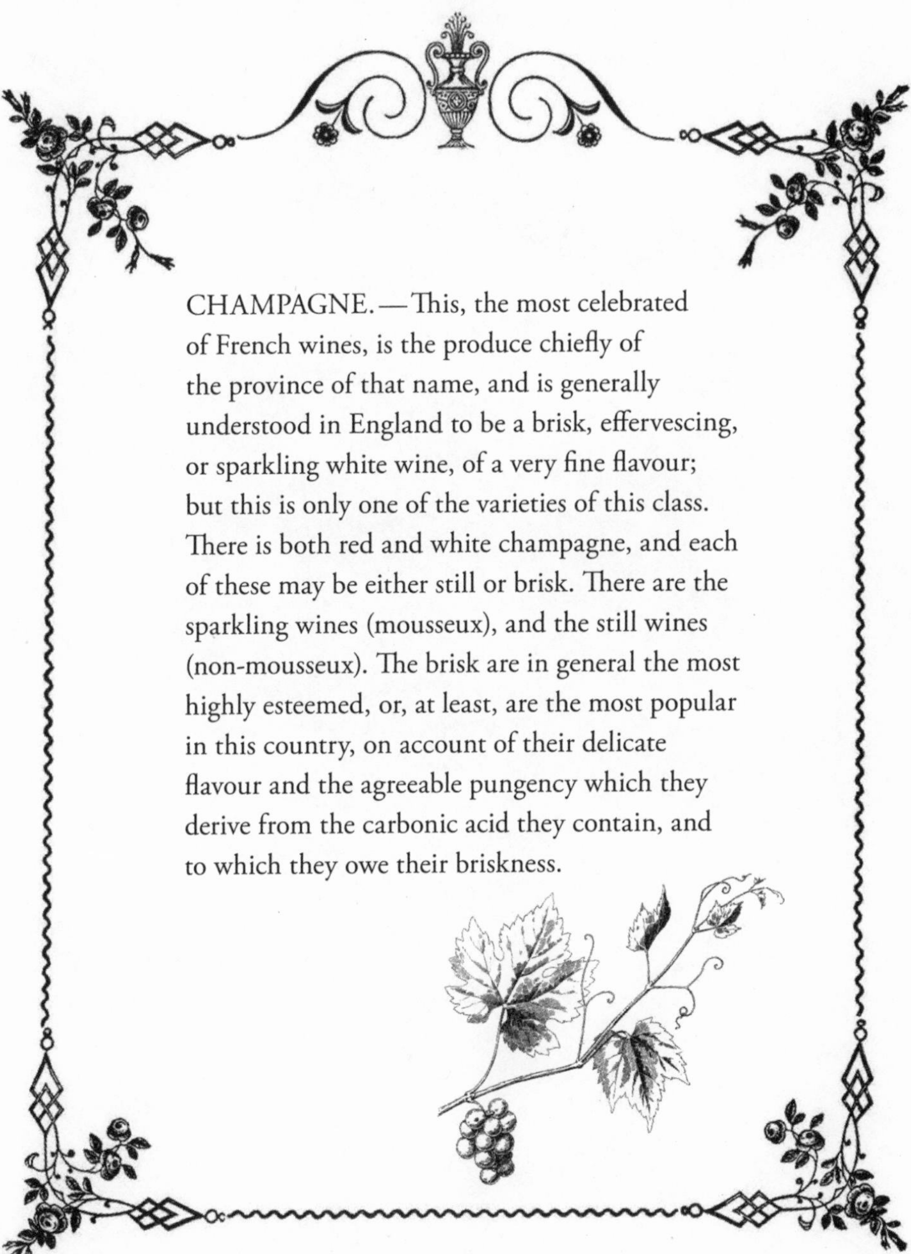

CHAMPAGNE.—This, the most celebrated of French wines, is the produce chiefly of the province of that name, and is generally understood in England to be a brisk, effervescing, or sparkling white wine, of a very fine flavour; but this is only one of the varieties of this class. There is both red and white champagne, and each of these may be either still or brisk. There are the sparkling wines (mousseux), and the still wines (non-mousseux). The brisk are in general the most highly esteemed, or, at least, are the most popular in this country, on account of their delicate flavour and the agreeable pungency which they derive from the carbonic acid they contain, and to which they owe their briskness.

CHAPTER FIFTEEN

Musing on the Theme of Union

1867–68

Following his arrival in England in late November, and in spite of all the talks, debates, dinners, drinking sessions, and even setting himself on fire, Macdonald had managed some other rather extraordinary business: he'd found himself a new wife. On February 16, 1867, John A. married Susan Agnes Bernard, a Jamaican-born Englishwoman twenty-one years his junior, at St. George's Church in London's Hanover Square.

They had first met one another in 1856, at the Rossin House Hotel in Toronto, where twenty-year-old Agnes was dining with her brother. Although he was married to Isabella, Macdonald made it his business to learn more about Agnes and her family. He learned that she was from a respectable English family that now lived on the shores of Lake Simcoe. Ever the strategist, within the year, John A. had hired Agnes's brother Hewitt as his private secretary, which helped facilitate inviting her to his Valentine's Day ball in Quebec City in 1860. John A. crossed paths with her at least once that night as he giddily handed out his valentines. Agnes was certainly interested in John A., if for no other reason than her interest in politics. She was worldly, intelligent, and attractive in a handsome sort of way, and yet John A. had several love interests at the time and was often surrounded by beautiful women, all admiring his wit and unable to resist the allure of so powerful a man.

The sudden wedding was a rather dramatic surprise. The proposal must have happened after his last letter home, dated December 27, 1866, since he made no mention of Agnes, an engagement, or a wedding. Given that he had been critical of the haste of his sister Margaret's wedding, one might have expected him to take some time to inform his family. There was a likely reason for all the haste. Macdonald's "dalliances" and general bad behaviour were attracting public attention, and since he was about to lead the colonies and provinces into confederation, a wife would be, for him, useful socially and likely a civilizing influence. Agnes was thirty-one years old, and so long as she was unmarried she had no status, no future, and was dependent on her family. Marrying John A. Macdonald, she would assume both prestige and a place in Canadian history. If not a passionate love affair, it was at least a strategic alliance for both of them.

The wedding was a pretty one, with rays of winter sunlight streaming in through the stained-glass windows of St. George's Church in fashionable Mayfair. Agnes wore white. The bridesmaids wore pastel dresses with matching bonnets. Macdonald gave a charming speech in which he mused on the theme of union. The ninety guests in attendance were treated by Agnes's brother to a sumptuous wedding breakfast at the Westminster Palace Hotel. There were bunches of snowdrops and violets at each place setting and, as the newspapers reported, "every known delicacy to eat." The happy couple left immediately for a short honeymoon in Oxford.

On February 19, 1867, just three days after the wedding, the British North America Bill was introduced to the House of Commons in Westminster. The bill sailed through its first and second readings and by March 8 had passed third reading. By the end of March, Queen Victoria granted Royal Assent. The British North America Act was now officially law and was set to take effect on July 1, 1867.

The newlyweds returned to Canada at the beginning of May, moving into John A.'s home on Daly Street in Ottawa, along with Agnes's mother, Theodora. Mere days after their return, on May 6, John A. joined his Cabinet colleagues for a celebratory lunch of cold beef and mutton at the

Rideau Club. By late afternoon he was carried out, hopelessly drunk, his vows to Agnes to curb, but not entirely quit his drinking, were all but forgotten.

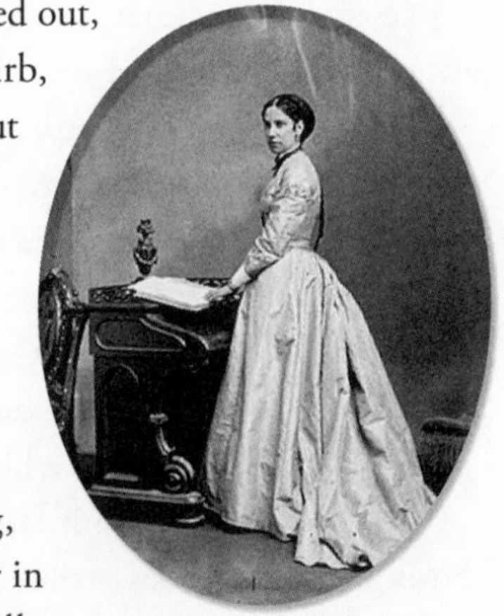

Susan Agnes Bernard Macdonald

With the exception of the Parliament buildings, Ottawa's Gothic architectural jewels, the city was little more than a rough logging town, notorious for both drunken brawls and an inadequate sewage system, the smell of which permeated everything, even the Macdonald home. At times, the air in their house was so foul that it made them ill. Between the scarce housing supply and John A.'s mounting debts, there was no hope of moving, so they had to stay put and endure it.

Their patience was well rewarded for, on the morning of July 1, 1867, Dominion Day, John A. received word that he had been granted a knighthood. He was now Sir John A. Macdonald, and Agnes, to her huge excitement, was Lady Macdonald. The new nation was born amongst much triumphant celebration and noise. All across the dominion church bells pealed and concert bands played, while picnics, parades, parties, cricket games, horse races, and military salutes took place. In the evening, there were bonfires and fireworks. In Ottawa the new Parliament Buildings were finally complete.

On July 5, Agnes wrote in her diary, "Now I am a great Premier's wife and Lady Macdonald and Cabinet secrets and mysteries might drop off… my pen."[48] For a few months, the great Premier's wife spent some happy days learning the ropes of her new job. When Parliament reconvened in November, she could often be found in the gallery, looking down on the proceedings. At times, she and John A. rode home together in a sleigh through the snow-lined streets.

One of Agnes's new responsibilities was to host afternoon tea and dinner parties. When the House was in session, every Saturday night a party of guests would arrive at their house, including members of Parliament and Cabinet ministers. In November she wrote in her diary, "We had a large dinner party last night—12—and everything was very nice indeed. John seemed in good spirits & so satisfied that I was ever so happy."[49] While that meal had gone off without a hitch, other occasions did go quite so smoothly.

She seemed particularly stumped by a visit from Hugh John, who took a break from his studies at the University of Toronto in January 1868 to make a rare visit to his father. Agnes organized a tea party in Hugh's honour, but unfortunately it wasn't to be one of her more successful attempts. John A. failed to turn up on time. And Agnes, nervous and unsure of herself, spilled the tea and failed to engage Hugh, writing in her diary, "Tea and games and supper, but it was very stupid, I could do nothing to promote gaiety."[50]

Agnes was not a particularly relaxed or imaginative hostess. She often wrote in her diary about her botched attempts at entertaining. It wasn't as though she had to cook—there were servants for that—but she was expected to plan the meals and be charming. Her taste in food ran to such uninspired dishes as mock-turtle soup, mutton, and apple pudding. After one evening of entertaining she wrote in her diary, "John says the dinner last night was a failure."[51] Her ability to make interesting small talk was almost non-existent. More often than not, as well-intentioned and intelligent as she was, Agnes could seem pious and rather critical.

AFTERNOON TEA WITH LADY AGNES

The Victorian tradition of afternoon tea was alive and well in the Dominion of Canada, where ladies often gathered in one another's homes for a formal afternoon tea. Larger, less formal afternoon teas, particularly those that included both men and women, were referred to as *kettle drums*.

The term derived from *tea kettle* and from *drum*, which was a very old name for a party. Typically teas were held late in the afternoon, around five o'clock. The menu was flexible but usually consisted of a selection of finger sandwiches, buns, plain or currant scones or tea cakes, small tarts, a cake, a variety of biscuits including macaroons, gingersnaps, and shortbread, and, of course, a large pot of tea.

Macaroons were very popular throughout the Victorian era. The earliest ones were made of almond paste, although later they were made with ground almonds and, later still, coconut. The following recipe from *Mrs. Beeton's Book of Household Management*, 1861, called for sweet almonds to be soaked and then pounded; ground almonds or almond meal could be easily substituted. Parchment can be used in place of wafer-paper.

Teacakes or scones were practically mandatory at afternoon tea. Both evolved from bannock: scones were made with baking soda (or similar), and teacakes were usually made with yeast.

Catharine Parr Traill's version of teacakes from *The Canadian Settlers' Guide* (originally published as *The Female Emigrant's Guide*) is more akin to a scone recipe. Traill was a naturalist and writer. She was born in England and came to Canada in 1832 with her husband. Two of her sisters, Agnes Strickland and Susanna Moodie, were also writers. Moodie moved to Canada, shortly after Traill, and the two sisters both wrote about pioneer life. Their books are among the richest sources of information about settler life in Upper Canada in the mid-1800s.

Traill's hot teacakes are best served warm with butter and jam.

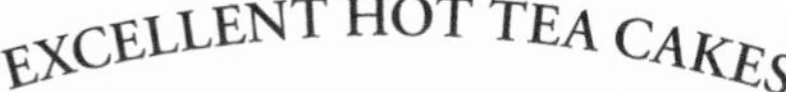

EXCELLENT HOT TEA CAKES

One quart of fine flour: two ounces of butter: two teaspoonfuls of cream of tartar, mixed dry through the flour: one teaspoonful of salaratus or soda: moisten the latter in milk or water till dissolved: mix with sweet milk or cold water.

These cakes to be rolled, and cut out with a tumbler, about an inch in thickness, served hot and buttered.

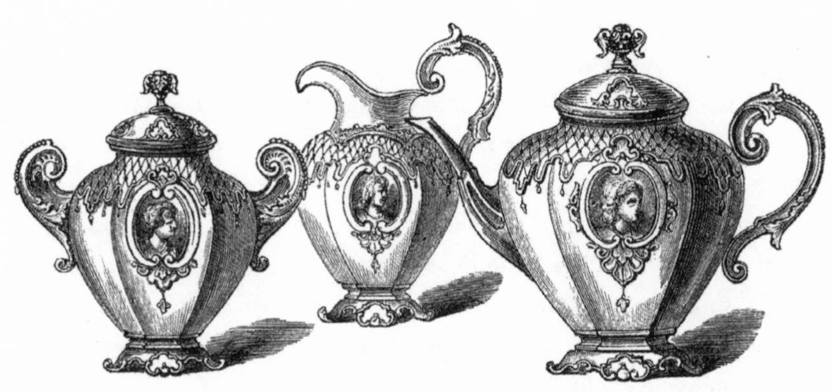

MACAROONS

1744. INGREDIENTS—1/2 lb. of sweet almonds, 1/2 lb. of sifted loaf sugar, the whites of 3 eggs, wafer-paper.

Mode.—Blanch, skin, and dry the almonds, and pound them well with a little orange-flower water or plain water; then add to them the sifted sugar and the whites of the eggs, which should be beaten to a stiff froth, and mix all the ingredients well together. When the paste looks soft, drop it at equal distances from a biscuit-syringe on to sheets of wafer-paper; put a strip of almond on the top of each; strew some sugar over, and bake the macaroons in rather a slow oven, of a light brown colour when hard and set, they are done, and must not be allowed to get very brown, as that would spoil their appearance. If the cakes, when baked, appear heavy, add a little more white of egg, but let this always be well whisked before it is added to the other ingredients. We have given a recipe for making these cakes, but we think it almost or quite as economical to purchase such articles as these at a good confectioner's.

Time.—From 15 to 20 minutes, in a slow oven.
Average cost, 1s. 8d. per lb.

CHAPTER SIXTEEN

A Roast Duck Dinner Saves the Dominion

1867–69

In October 1867, the Commercial Bank collapsed and very nearly took Macdonald down with it. The bank, based in Kingston, had been overextended for years, having had a run of bad luck with unreliable borrowers. One, in particular, the Right Honourable Sir John A. Macdonald, owed the bank in excess of $80,000, ten times his salary as prime minister and an astronomical amount of money in its time. The failure of the bank had far-reaching consequences for Macdonald: he was perilously close to personal bankruptcy, and given that the bank was in his home riding of Kingston, he was fast losing political points. As a final straw, he lost his finance minister, Galt, who resigned in exasperation over the bank's failure.

Meanwhile there were larger political issues to be concerned with, because the administrative mechanisms of the old union were quite unsuited to the new federal needs. An interprovincial railway was needed to link Ontario and Quebec with the Maritimes. At the same time, the United States had cancelled the Reciprocity Treaty in 1866, limiting the free flow of Canadian goods such as fish, timber, and agricultural products into the US. In addition, new annexation threats started to arise in the Northwest Territories. In the east, Prince Edward Island and Newfoundland refused to join the Confederation, and Nova Scotia was making fresh noises about leaving—a threat which if carried out would destabilize the future of the nation. In short, far from solving all of the new Dominion of Canada's problems, confederation was the beginning of a lot of new ones. It was an extremely trying time.

In November 1867, Parliament resumed and Macdonald began by forming a Cabinet, a delicate juggling process fraught with infighting, backstabbing, and raging jealousy. On December 10, a Customs Bill was introduced which would have serious consequences for New Brunswick and Nova Scotia, not the least of which was an increased duty on spirits entering Canada. In Ontario and Quebec, domestic Canadian rye whisky was the drink of choice, but Maritimers favoured imported rum and brandy, and the new customs duties affected them disproportionately. Finance Minister John Rose told the Maritimers to suck it up and learn to drink Upper Canadian rye. The Maritimers were furious. It was a small but important issue, one to which Sir John, of all people, should have been sympathetic.

All the talk of liquor drove Macdonald back to the bottle. One month later, in January 1868, Agnes gave up wine in an attempt to set an appropriate example. John A. scarcely noticed and paid her no heed whatsoever. By now a new problem had arisen. Their cesspit had frozen, and the house was swamped with the odour of raw sewage that had nowhere to go.

In February 1868, with Nova Scotia seriously threatening to pull out of confederation, Macdonald considered quitting politics again, an idea he had contemplated nearly as often as he moved house. His friends told him he should join the judicial bench, but he rejected this outright, proclaiming that he would rather go straight to hell.

The real breaking point came on April 7, 1868, when Macdonald's trusted colleague, drinking partner, and old friend D'Arcy McGee was brutally murdered in the middle of the night. John A. was shattered. It seems he sobered up long enough to find comfort in the arms of Agnes, because only a few weeks later, she announced that she was pregnant.

It was Nova Scotia though, that dominated the political agenda. Determined to extract themselves from confederation, they went so far as to send their anti-confederation former premier, Joseph Howe, to London, England, to plead for Nova Scotia's release from the British North America Act. To counter Howe's arguments, Macdonald sent his old chum Charles Tupper, one of the Fathers of Confederation and also a former Nova Scotia premier, off to London to argue the necessity of keeping Nova Scotia in the dominion.

London ruled that confederation was a fixed fact. This brought new fears that Nova Scotia might try to join the United States or simply seek independence. In August 1868, anti-confederation members of the dominion met in Nova Scotia for a convention to investigate their options. John A. assembled a delegation to attend and brought a pregnant Agnes along as well. Macdonald's mission was to offer a conciliatory presence, a balanced viewpoint, and practical remedies, including the possibility of federal funds for Nova Scotia. The gestures were vital to the future of the country. Without Nova Scotia in the union, there might well have been disastrous consequences for the Dominion of Canada.

Amongst all the politics and problems, life went on. On New Year's Day 1869, Sir John and Lady Agnes welcomed over ninety guests to their annual New Year's Day Levee. Agnes, eight months pregnant, was in her glory as the guests crowded into their Daly Street home. The attendees drank sherry and champagne and made their way through bowls of oyster soup and a spread of hot and cold canapés. Agnes wrote in her diary, "Visiting began soon after noon and I had such a busy day, pleasant day. Luncheon going on from then till 5:30 and about 90 callers. I like so much this old-fashioned custom — it is so truly kind and cordial and friendly — my husband helped me and so did my dear old mother and we all enjoyed ourselves."[52]

Less than one month later, a triumphant and heavily pregnant Agnes, buoyed by her pregnancy and her successful New Year's party, organized a dinner for Joseph Howe, the disgruntled Nova Scotian who had the led the charge against confederation. Plied with wine and roast duck,[53] Howe and Macdonald negotiated the financial deal for Nova Scotia that Macdonald had first mentioned at the Halifax convention the previous summer. In return, Howe confirmed Nova Scotia's commitment to confederation. Macdonald sealed the deal by offering Howe a position in the Cabinet.

Soothed by dinner and seduced by money and the prospect of a Cabinet position, Howe and therefore Nova Scotia were once again committed to confederation, and the Dominion of Canada remained intact. Agnes's roast duck dinner had saved the nation.

NEW YEAR'S LEVEES AND POWER DINNERS IN THE 1800s

The New Year's Levee is a distinctly Canadian event: elsewhere in the world, a *levée* generally means a formal reception given by the sovereign or a representative, usually only for male invitees. In fact, the term's origin stems from the court of Louis XIV, who met male subjects in his chambers, at sunrise. In Canada the event was associated with New Year's Day festivities, beginning with the governor of New France's levee in Quebec City on January 1, 1646. Subsequently, the fur traders adopted the tradition of paying their respects to their government representatives on New Year's Day, and the custom was taken up by British colonial governors and spread to include levees held by high-ranking military officials and elected representatives.

There are many references to New Year's levees at the various homes of John A. The house would have been decorated with garlands of greenery and ribbons for Christmas, which were taken down on the evening of January 5, preceding Twelfth Day or Epiphany, the last day of Christmas festivities in the Christian faith. Unlike the formal levees held by foreign sovereigns and their representatives, New Year's levees in Canada were lively events for everyone. They generally began around noon and went on until early evening. Levees were important social events and invitations were highly prized.

As well as plenty of sherry, wine, and champagne, there was almost always a large pot of oyster soup, along with platters of roast beef, chicken, ham, and turkey. Sometimes there were dressed mutton chops. There would also have been a variety of breads, cooked vegetables, and desserts.

Over the years, Agnes recorded various different remarks about the Macdonald New Year's Levees in her diary. In 1871 she wrote:

> *What a bustling day this has been! All the fires blazing and crackling, the house in its best order, all the servants important and in a hurry and I in my best black velveteen gown, receiving New Year's visitors! The house was thronged from noon til dinner time, with men of all ages, sorts, and styles. Some 130 in all—some merely shook hands or bowed, exchanged a few commonplaces about the weather, but the larger part lunched at a continually replenished table in the dining room and wished me and mine all the happiness of the New Year between mouthfuls of hot oyster soup or sips of sherry.*[54]

The Macdonalds' weekly dinner parties were legendary, and for most who attended, the dinners were an intoxicating and seductive mixture of power, politics, alcohol, food and lively, meaningful, and often witty conversation. Although Agnes had initially struggled with her social responsibilities, she was quick and willing to learn. Though she needed John A.'s conversational abilities and gaiety to keep things lively, through sheer volume alone, she learned the skills necessary to plan and execute a successful party and had become adept at choosing appealing and stylish menus.

Duck was a perfect dinner party choice. Both wild and domesticated ducks were relatively abundant but not deemed as commonplace as pork or chicken. Often served with a port or currant sauce, duck was considered fashionable. Ducks were also valued for their feathers and giblets. The giblets were a favourite for making stocks and gravies.

Oysters were another remarkably popular and fashionable food. Shop owners, hoteliers, and tavern keepers went to great lengths to have supplies on hand throughout the year. Oysters, packed live in barrels, were transported by boat and stagecoach before rail lines existed. During the winter months supplies of oysters were buried in beds of damp sand mixed with cornmeal and watered routinely. By the mid-1800s canned oysters were available but because of a lack of proper sterilization techniques and subsequent blood poisoning, the early shellfish canning industry did not survive.

Used in soups, stews, and curries, oysters were also served fried, roasted, boiled, pickled, creamed, skewered, and made into patties, croquettes, fritters, and pies. By the late 1800s, the North American love affair with oysters was such that the eastern beds began to be depleted.

Oyster soup was not just for New Year's levees; it also featured regularly as a starter at dinner parties in the Macdonald household. Recipes for oyster soup (*The Canadian Home Cook Book,* 1877), roast duck, and currant sauce (both from *The Canadian Housewife's Manual of Cookery*) follow.

OYSTER SOUP

Take one quart of water, one teacup of butter; one pint of milk, two teaspoons of salt, four crackers rolled fine, and one teaspoon of pepper; bring to full boiling heat as soon as possible, then add one quart of oysters; let the whole come to boiling heat quickly and remove from fire.

DUCKS, ROASTED

13. Stuff one with sage and onion, a dessert spoonful of crumbs, a bit of butter, and pepper and salt; let the other be unseasoned. Serve with a fine gravy.

THE OLD CURRANT SAUCE

23. Boil an ounce of dried currants in half a pint of water for a few minutes; then add a small tea-cupful of breadcrumbs, six cloves, a glass of port wine, and a bit of butter. Stir it 'til the whole is smooth.

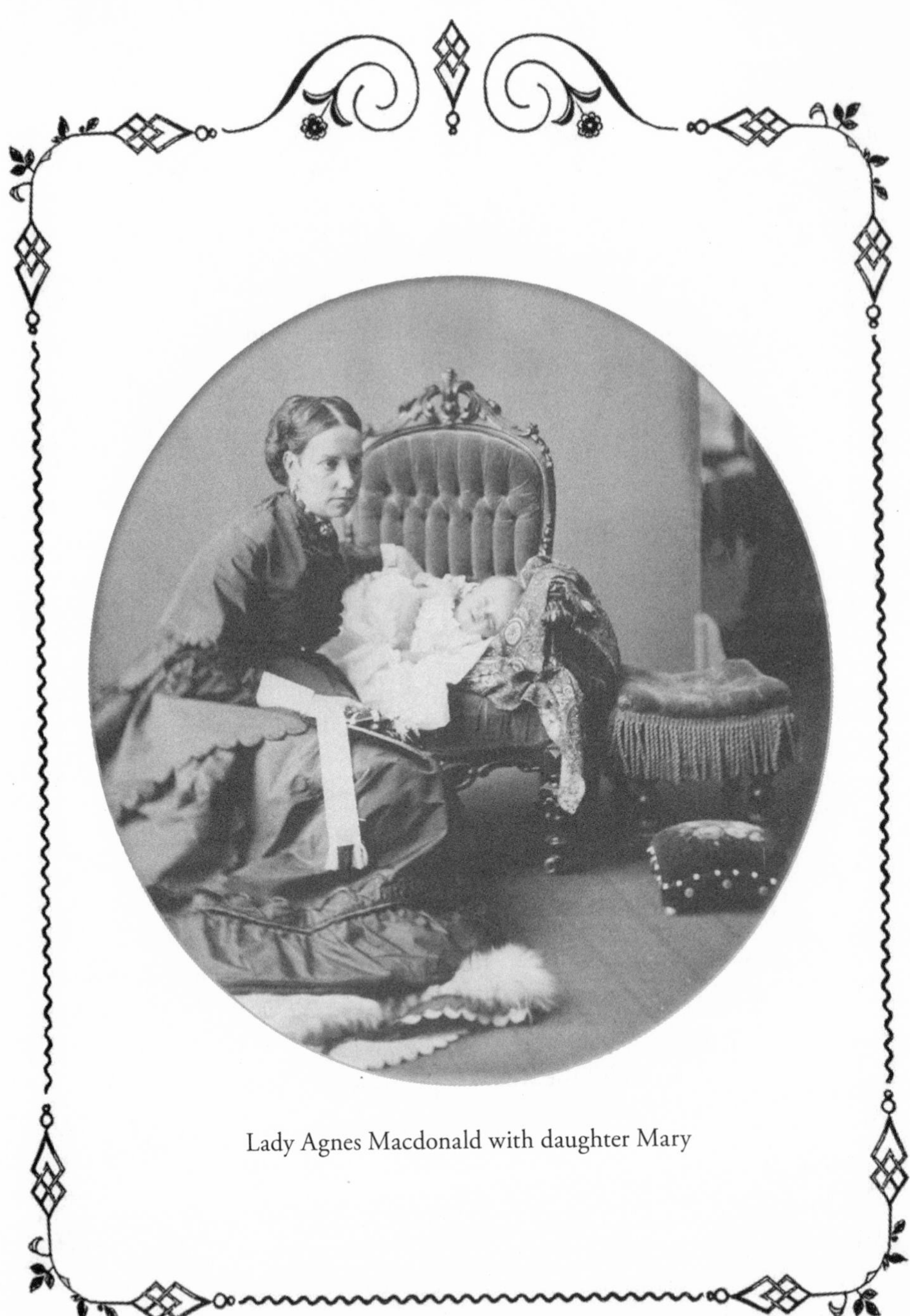

Lady Agnes Macdonald with daughter Mary

CHAPTER SEVENTEEN

The Hopes of the Nation Hang on Half an Oyster

1869–70

On February 8, 1869, Mary Theodora Macdonald entered the world after a long and arduous labour. Her parents were ecstatic. Agnes recorded in her diary, "She is laying asleep in her blankets — my very own darling baby — my little daughter, the sweet gift from Heaven, my Mary — a dark-eyed, soft thing. What word can tell how my heart swells with love and pride — she is truly dear."[55]

Shortly after delivery, Mary was diagnosed with the condition known as hydrocephalus, or water on the brain. It was thought that her life would be short, and it was not known if she would ever walk or talk or be able to look after herself. Agnes was clearly heartbroken but if John A. was depressed over the news, he never showed it. It is perhaps one of the most telling aspects of his character that he developed a profound, fierce, protective, and unconditional love for his Little Baboo, as he called Mary, and he treated her as though she were a princess and spent time with her daily, regardless of what else was going on in his life.

In April the same year, while he was still reeling from the birth of his disabled daughter, the Montreal bank overseeing Macdonald's finances called in his debt. He had no choice but to sell off his properties. Aged fifty-four years, with a seriously handicapped baby daughter whose future was entirely uncertain, Macdonald now had precious little left but his modest salary. As was typical of his routine, he escaped into the bottle and yet still carried on with governing the country.

After a difficult series of negotiations in London, Canada purchased the territorial rights of the Hudson's Bay Company, the land known as Rupert's Land, for £300,000. In fact, the United States had been eyeing this land since, after acquiring Alaska from the Russians in March 1867 for $7.2 million, it was still looking to expand. The US felt that owning this large piece of the North American continent was its manifest destiny and made an offer of $10 million to the Hudson's Bay Company. Macdonald, however, was determined that this territory, which included what are now the three prairie provinces, as well as most of northern Ontario and Quebec and part of Labrador, should belong to the Dominion of Canada.

The land purchase was fundamental in Macdonald's vision of a great nation from sea to sea. However, the deal ignored the First Nations and Métis peoples. The Red River colony was home to 11,000 inhabitants, including First Nations, French-speaking Métis, English-speaking Métis, Hudson's Bay Company employees, and immigrants from Ontario and the United States, many of whom had no wish to become Canadians.

Macdonald appointed Ontario Liberal William McDougall as the lieutenant-governor of the Northwest Territories. McDougall set out for the Red River settlement to establish his authority. Just below the 49th parallel, in a small town south of Winnipeg, McDougall ran into trouble. His way was blocked and a note advised him that "The National Committee of the Métis of Red River instruct Mr. McDougall not to enter the Northwest Territory without special permission from this Committee." It was signed by John Bruce and Louis Riel. Riel had established a provisional government with the goal of resisting annexation by the Dominion of Canada.

In failing to recognize the importance of the Métis, and in treating Louis Riel as a rebel because he was leading the resistance against joining the

Dominion of Canada, John A. set in motion a series of events that could be described as one of the greatest blunders in his political career. Hoping for a peaceful settlement, he sent a second emissary, Donald Smith, to the territory. Things did not go as planned. A number of prisoners were taken. One of them, Thomas Scott, was convicted and jailed for rebelling against the Riel government. Scott was sentenced to death and executed by a Métis firing squad on March 4, 1870. There were rumours that he was still alive when he was placed in his coffin. This provoked Ontario Protestants, and soon the anger expanded as French Canadians came to Louis Riel's defence. Now Quebec and Ontario were firmly pitted against each other, and the furor showed no signs of abating.

Riel demanded that the Red River Colony become a full province in its own right within the Dominion of Canada. Macdonald was prepared to acquiesce, primarily because he recognized that without the Red River Colony, soon to become the province of Manitoba, further westward expansion would be difficult. In the spring of 1870, Macdonald sent an Anglo-Canadian military expedition to the Red River to bring about the annexation of the Northwest Territories. As the expedition approached, Riel fled into exile and annexation of the territories proceeded.

In Ottawa, Parliament waited for the prime minister to table legislation to create the new province of Manitoba, but he did not appear. There were reports that he was unwell. The *Globe* immediately cried foul, claiming Macdonald was on yet another almighty drinking spree. It ran a story with the headline "A Foul Disgrace."[56] From all reports it seemed that he had been inebriated throughout the entire period.

On May 6, 1870, Macdonald was in his office in the East Block on Parliament Hill when Hewitt Bernard, his assistant, heard a crash. He entered Macdonald's office and found the prime minister in convulsions, writhing on the floor, his pulse almost undetectable. In the hours that followed, it appeared that Macdonald was dying. A telegram was dispatched to Hugh John to let him know about his father's condition. The pain was so severe that Macdonald did not even recognize Agnes, who rushed to be at his side. A doctor was summoned, morphine was administered, and John A. was diagnosed with gallstones. Gallbladder surgery was not yet a possibility so those suffering with acute cholecystitis—a blocked and swollen gallbladder—had no choice but to endure the pain and hope the gallstones would pass. For a month John A. remained in his office on Parliament Hill, now converted to a sickroom.

In the meantime, Parliament adjourned but not before the Manitoba Act had proceeded and Royal Assent was quickly received.

Hugh John came to visit. Agnes, who despaired of John A.'s drinking, took to rubbing her husband's chest and face with whiskey to soothe him. Even the *Globe* softened its attacks and reported that Sir John was "very low." There were genuine fears and concerns that the nation might lose its leader. Public sympathy was high.

Dr. James Grant, John A.'s physician, put Macdonald on a diet of poached white fish and milk and reminded him how ill he had been and how risky it would be to over indulge. He told John A. that he could have just half an oyster as a treat. "Remember, Sir John," said Dr. Grant, "The hopes of Canada are now depending on you."

"It seems strange," replied John A., "that the hopes of Canada should depend on half an oyster."[57]

THE SICK ROOM

During the 1800s doctors were few and far between, especially in rural areas where many could not afford a doctor even if one was available. Physicians had only rudimentary remedies for treating illnesses. Essentially all they could do was treat pain and suffering. Penicillin, for example, was not discovered until 1928 and not in use until the 1940s. Insulin was not discovered until 1921 at the University of Toronto. Heroin, morphine, cannabis, and laudanum (opium mixed with alcohol) were widely available and routinely used to treat children and adults suffering with anything from pain, coughs, colds, and toothaches to more serious illnesses such as cancer and liver disease. Of these drugs, opium and its derivative morphine were the most commonly used. Unfortunately, both were highly addictive and could have long-term, life-changing effects. But many are surprised that cannabis was also widely used. "Even Queen Victoria was prescribed tincture of cannabis," the journalist Steven Poole notes. "It is believed she was amused."[58]

Much of the care of sick patients was provided by family members since there was not yet a medical establishment with hospitals and nurses. Almost all cookbooks and emigrant's guides of the era have substantial sections on treating the elderly and infirm. These passages make interesting reading. In addition to traditional medicines, a variety of homemade treatments were used for a range of illnesses including fever and ague, caked breast, wasp and bee stings, cholera, swollen glands, constipation, smallpox, hydrophobia, corns, felon (infections of the fingertip pulp), hoarseness, sore throat, eruptive disease, toothache, headache, chilblains, hysteria, and "summer complaint."

Broths, including beef tea, calf's foot broth, and eel broth were popular in the sick room, as were gruels, pastes, and tinctures. *Mrs. Beeton* offered a comprehensive section on homeopathic medicine and homeopathic remedies and an entire section of the book, "Invalid Cookery," included recipes for toast water, white wine whey, and barley gruel.

Some of the more interesting treatments from a variety of sources are given here.

TO EXPEL NAMELESS INTRUDERS FROM CHILDREN'S HEADS

(from *The Cook Not Mad*)

Steep larkspur seed in water, rub the liquor a few times into the child's hair and the business of destruction is done. This is an effectual remedy. Does it not make your head itch?

ARTIFICIAL ASSES MILK

(from *The Canadian Housewife's Manual of Cookery*)

36. Boil together a quart of water, a quart of new milk, an ounce of white sugar-candy, half an ounce of eringo-root, and half an ounce of conserve of roses, till half be wasted. This is astringent; therefore proportion the doses to the effect, and the quantity to what will be used while sweet.

FOR A CAKED BREAST—A HIGHLAND REMEDY

(from *The Canadian Home Cook Book*, 1877)

Bake large potatoes, put two or more in a woolen stocking; crush them soft and apply to the breast as hot as can be borne; repeat constantly till relieved.

—Mrs. G.B. Wyllie.

GRAVEL OR SAND IN URINE

(from *Mrs. Beeton's Book of Household Management*, 1861)

Gravel or sand in the urine is due to an excess of uric acid in the system.

A gouty tendency, too much rich food, and a sluggish liver will cause the excess.

Treatment consists in adopting a plain, light and spare diet, avoiding sweets, creams, wines, malt liquors and much red meat, and in taking plenty of demulcent drinks, such as barley-water or milk and soda. A dose of Carlsbad salts in the morning, with a mild mercurial pill over night will relieve the congested liver.

FROST-BITE

(from *Mrs. Beeton's Book of Household Management,* 1861)

Parts most frequently affected: ears, nose, cheeks, fingers and toes. The frost bitten part is greyish-white, and absolutely insensitive. Treatment. Rub with snow or ice-cold water till sensation returns.

Artificial warmth applied to a frost-bite will cause mortification.

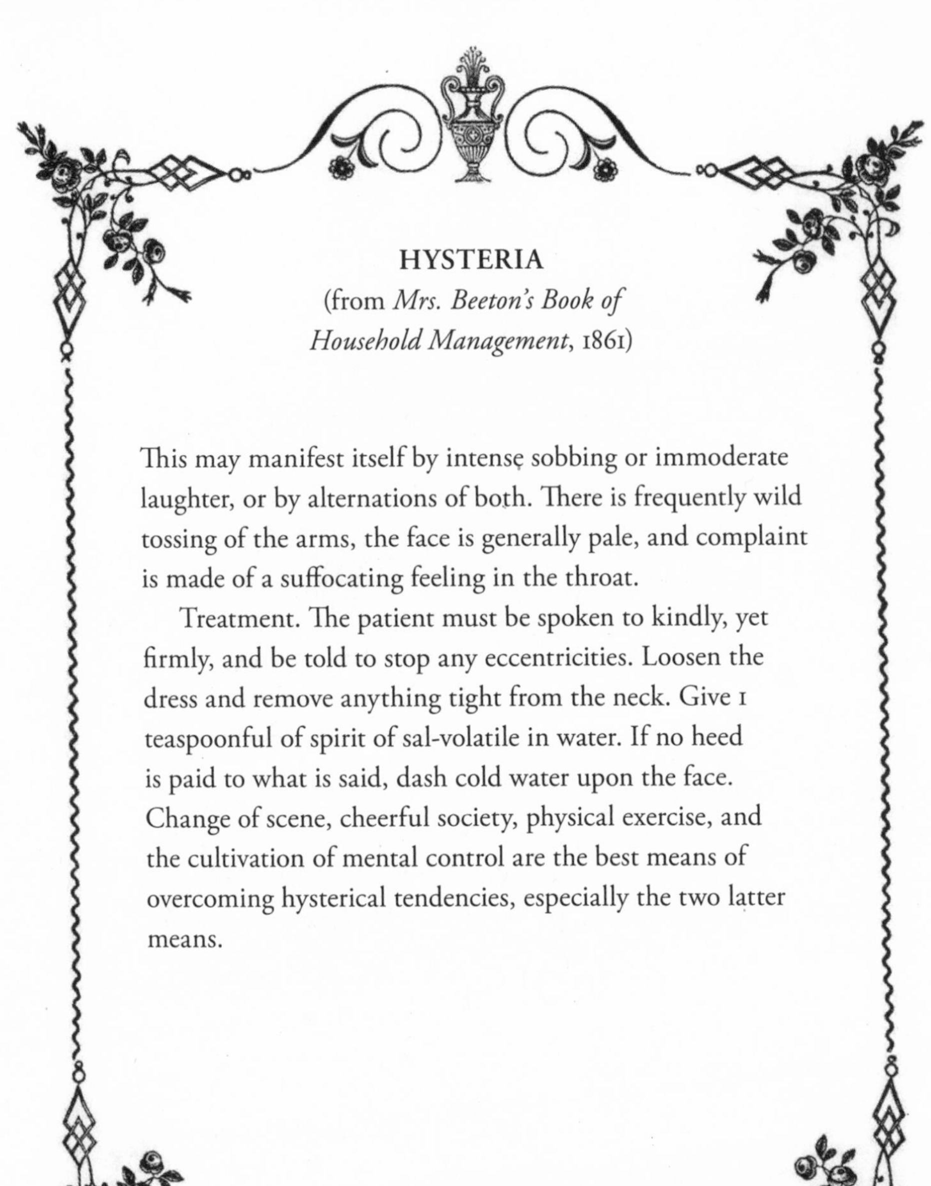

HYSTERIA

(from *Mrs. Beeton's Book of Household Management*, 1861)

This may manifest itself by intense sobbing or immoderate laughter, or by alternations of both. There is frequently wild tossing of the arms, the face is generally pale, and complaint is made of a suffocating feeling in the throat.

Treatment. The patient must be spoken to kindly, yet firmly, and be told to stop any eccentricities. Loosen the dress and remove anything tight from the neck. Give 1 teaspoonful of spirit of sal-volatile in water. If no heed is paid to what is said, dash cold water upon the face. Change of scene, cheerful society, physical exercise, and the cultivation of mental control are the best means of overcoming hysterical tendencies, especially the two latter means.

CHAPTER EIGHTEEN

The Pacific Scandal and Time Off to Feed the Chickens

1870–73

Macdonald was still ill in bed when British Columbia agreed to become the sixth province. Transformed by the gold rush of 1858 but isolated from the rest of the Dominion, British Columbia had become another possible target of American annexation. In June 1870, George-Étienne Cartier, who was at the helm during Macdonald's illness, negotiated the terms of union. Canada would ensure that British Columbia, heavily in debt, was financially stable and that within a decade there would be a transcontinental railway, linking the dominion from the Atlantic Ocean to the Pacific. Cartier had just committed Canada, with its population of only four million, to building the world's longest railway system.

By July, Macdonald was well enough to leave his sick bed and continue his convalescence in Prince Edward Island. He had a motive other than just the good sea air. PEI was not yet part of the union and Macdonald wanted to make his presence known. It took another three years, but finally Prince Edward Island became the seventh province to join the dominion, in a quiet and unassuming manner, on July 1, 1873.

John A. and his family spent a happy summer in PEI before returning to Ottawa in mid-September 1870. Once back, they moved into a new, bigger home, called Earnscliffe. For a few months, the Macdonalds enjoyed a semblance of normality while they set up home.

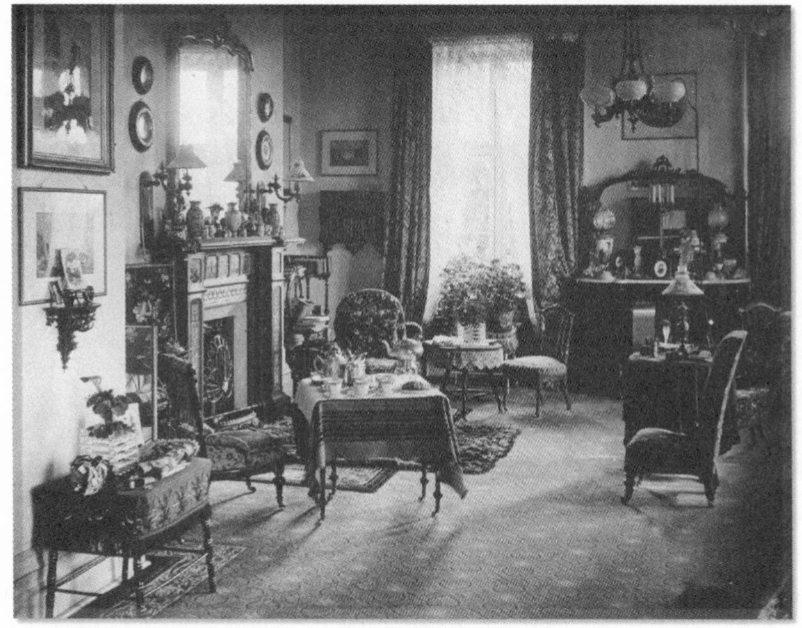

Drawing Room at Earnscliffe—The Table is Set for Tea

Hugh John had come home to help his father and family move, but the father-son relationship, damaged by many years of virtual estrangement, was volatile. John A. encouraged his son to follow in his footsteps and study the law. A reluctant Hugh John did decide to attend law school but only after some arguments with his father. The young Macdonald complained to his friends that Ottawa was boring and Agnes was overbearing. There are hints that John A. might have agreed on this point, although he simply did as he pleased. In a letter to a friend, Hugh John wrote about the many rules, claiming that he could not have his pals over or set off firecrackers and complaining of other seemingly trivial matters. "I had a great battle about smoking downstairs but I told them [Agnes and father] that if I could not smoke downstairs I would take my book up to my own room and smoke and read there. This they did not consider wholesome so they at last gave in and now I puff away in the dining room."[59]

Hugh John's return to Toronto likely suited the whole family, though he was said to have found difficulty locating "medically reliable scarlet women" there. He and his friends were apparently fond of the verse:

> Mary Mother, we believe
> That without sin you did conceive;
> Teach we pray thee us, believing,
> How to sin without conceiving.[60]

In the meantime, unbeknownst to John A., his loyal friends and supporters had pitched in to form a trust fund so that on his death there would be something for his family—something other than a financial hole. A total amount of $69,062.52 was deposited to a testimonial trust, under the terms that John A. could not touch the money himself, since his record in managing money was the very reason the trust was required.

Although he had much to catch up on after his illness, early in 1871, after their New Year's Levee, John A. and Agnes travelled to Washington to negotiate matters of mutual concern, most notably the fisheries. They left baby Mary behind in the company of a nurse. Macdonald was loath to leave Canada but, nevertheless, they spent almost three months in Washington, where they quickly wearied of the endless partying. In her biography of Sir John, Patricia Phenix quotes him as noting, "We are overwhelmed by hospitalities which we cannot refuse." Lord de Grey, the British delegate, agreed, writing: "Our life is rendered very intolerable by the endless feasts. We work all day and dine all night."[61] Macdonald found the whole process entirely disagreeable but saw no way out.

At the end of his stay, he pressured Britain to provide a "liberal offer" to ratify the proposed American agreement allowing the Americans to buy offshore fishing rights along the Canadian coast. The British agreed. The multi-million dollar loan from the British was also enough to launch the railway. Despite all the issues, Macdonald had simultaneously appeased the British, the Americans, and his fellow countrymen. He reluctantly signed the Treaty of Washington, telling himself and a colleague, "There go the fisheries."[62] Essentially he had just sold the rights to the fisheries for at least a portion of the new railway.

During the 1872 election campaign, Macdonald secured funds for the railway from two business men, Sir Hugh Allan of Montreal's Merchant Bank, and David MacPherson of Toronto. Macdonald proposed to form a company represented by both Allan and MacPherson and then commission the company with the building of the railway. Both men wanted the directorship of the new railway company, but Hugh Allan wanted it badly enough that he made substantial donations to both Macdonald and Cartier's election campaigns. The money was accepted, and most of it was then promptly spent bribing voters in one of the most unethical election campaigns in history. At one point, Macdonald sent an urgent telegram to Sir Hugh stating "Immediate, private. I must have another ten thousand—will be the last time of calling. Do not fail me; answer today." Hugh Allen's lawyer replied the same day, "Draw on me for ten thousand dollars."[63] These telegrams became a crucial piece of evidence in the Pacific Scandal and some of the most damning documents in Canadian political history.

In the end, Macdonald won his seat in Kingston by only 131 votes. Throughout Ontario, the results were similar. It was a narrow win—scarcely a victory at all. George-Étienne Cartier lost his Montreal East seat, and to add insult to injury, he was seriously ill with Bright's disease, a chronic and acute condition of the kidneys.

Immediately after the election, Macdonald turned all his attention to the matter of the promised railway. It was an unimaginable task. Great swathes of uninhabited and virtually impassable land had to be surveyed. There were lakes, rivers, gorges, and vast prairies to contend with. There were mountain ranges, dense scrub, and terrific forests. There were the long harsh winter months and the heat, mosquitoes, and blackflies of summer. The manpower required was not available, and the expense alone made the task almost insurmountable.

Sir Hugh Allan had donated so generously to the election campaign that he was assured of being appointed director of the new railway company. Macdonald had at first agreed but later retracted because he heard that Allan was set to sell control to American railway interests. Then, shortly after Parliament opened, on April 2, 1873, Lucius Seth Huntington, Liberal member of Parliament for Shefford, rocked the House of Commons with the allegation that the Canadian Pacific Railway project had been sold for campaign funds. Macdonald denied the accusation. Nonetheless, the Pacific Scandal, as it came to be known, dominated the Canadian newspapers and all proceedings in the House. The *Globe* ran the headline "The Story of the Pacific Scandal! A Ten-Column Broadsheet." One could practically sense George Brown's glee as he revealed that Sir Hugh had given the Conservative Party $179,000, a huge sum, for campaign expenses and in return had been promised the charter to build a new railway. Macdonald continued his simultaneous campaigns of denial and binge drinking.

The following month, Macdonald was devastated when news reached him that George-Étienne Cartier had died in England, where he had gone to seek treatment. When Macdonald received the news by a trans-Atlantic telegram delivered to him in the House of Commons, he was overcome by tears and unable to speak. He took the loss of his much-trusted political partner hard. Without Cartier at his side, he was left alone to deal with the Pacific Scandal and the overwhelming prospect of building a national railway. Never again in his political life did Macdonald form such a strong political partnership with any other leader.

One small bit of news softened the blow of Cartier's death temporarily.

Three days after Cartier's death, on May 23, 1873, Queen Victoria, acting on the advice of John A., approved the act to establish the North West Mounted Police, later to become the Royal Canadian Mounted Police, one of the most iconic of all Canadian institutions. The police were needed to bring law and order to, assert sovereignty over, and stop the free flow of American whiskey into the Northwest Territories. Their presence was necessary if a railroad was to encourage settlers to the West. At least temporarily, Macdonald was preoccupied with the establishment of the new police force.

After Cartier's funeral in June, Lady Agnes and Sir John travelled to Rivière-du-Loup for a brief summer holiday before Parliament was scheduled to resume on August 13. It was here, in Rivière-du-Loup, early in the morning on August 3, that he disappeared and went missing for two days. The *Montreal Witness* reported that John A. Macdonald had attempted suicide by jumping from the wharf. The *Globe* followed suit, only later issuing a vague correction. The truth is not known, but what is known is that Macdonald, plagued by worries and sorrow and the pressure of public life, went missing for two entire days and nobody, including Macdonald himself, seemed to know anything of his whereabouts during the time he was absent.

By mid-August, John A. was back in Ottawa, prepared to defend his own and his party's honour. Parliament, however, was prorogued until October 23. Macdonald took time to keep in touch with daughter Mary, who remained in Rivière-du-Loup for the rest of the summer in the care of Agnes's mother. In light of all the worry and trouble in his life, the letter is particularly touching.

Ottawa, August 25, 1873

My dearest Mary

You must know that your kind Mamma and I are very anxious to see you and Granny again. We have put a new carpet in your room and got everything ready for you.

The garden looks lovely just now. It is full of beautiful flowers and I hope you will see them before they are withered.

There are some fine melons in the garden. You must pick them for dinner and feed the chickens with the rind. You remember that Mamma cut my hair and made me look like a cropped donkey. It has grown quite long again. When you come home, you must not pull it too hard.

Give my love to dear good Grand Mamma and give her a kiss for me.

Give my love to Sarah too, and so good bye my pet and come home soon to your loving papa

John A.[64]

Meanwhile sleazy details of corruption and bribery from the election campaign continued to emerge. Both Liberals and Conservatives were involved, with the Liberal Party stealing documents and bribing clerks with exorbitant sums to procure evidence about the Conservatives' conduct.

John A. was now so permanently drunk that Senator Alexander Campbell, a former colleague, said, "I am very much afraid that he has kept himself more or less under the influence of wine, and that he really has no clear recollection of what he did on many occasions.... A night of excess always leaves a morning of nervous incapacity and we were subjected to this pain amongst others."[65]

On Monday November 3, 1873, a haggard and visibly shaken Macdonald showed up in the House. By evening, he had made one the most famous speeches of his life. Fortified by tumblers of neat gin disguised as water, Macdonald delivered a five-hour oration in front of a full and rapt House with visitors, including British prime minister Benjamin Disraeli and Lady Dufferin, the wife of governor general. He was almost contrite, saying,

> I have fought the battle of Confederation, the battle of union, the battle of dominion. I throw myself upon this House; I throw myself upon this country; I throw myself upon posterity; and I believe, and I know, that, notwithstanding the many failings in my life, I shall have the voice of this country, and this House, rallying around me.[66]

To the end he claimed that while funds had been received, there had not been a corrupt bargain and nothing had been promised to Sir Hugh Allan. The majority of Macdonald's many biographers tend to concur. Macdonald also claimed that campaign funds were received by both sides of the House. Again, he was probably correct.

At the conclusion of this marathon of speeches, he said:

> I leave it with this House with every confidence. I am equal to either fortune. I can see past the decision of this House either for or against me, but whether it be against me or for me, I know, and it is no vain boast to say so, for even my enemies will admit that I am no boaster, that there does not exist in Canada a man who has given more of his time, more of his heart, more of his wealth, or more of his intellect and power, such as it may be, for the good of this Dominion of Canada.[67]

Despite his rousing and triumphant speech, two days later, on November 5, 1873, Macdonald officially resigned as prime minister, stating that he needed a rest and that he believed Canada would do him justice in the long run. To this day, he remains the only Canadian prime minister ever forced out of office by a scandal. When he returned home to Agnes that evening he was no longer the prime minister and she no longer the great Premier's wife. Whether he meant it or not, he told her, "Well, that's got along with. The Government has resigned. It's a relief to be out of it."[68]

ABOUT THOSE CHICKENS

Following his resignation, John A. had time for tending the chickens—the ones that he had written about in the letter to Mary. This was one of many references he made to the family having a garden plot and keeping poultry. Those who were able, in town or country, kept a few chickens and grew whatever vegetables they could. Food scraps, leftovers, and peelings that could not be used to make stock were fed to the chickens who returned the favour in eggs and eventually, roast fowl.

A Gentlewoman in Upper Canada includes a letter Anne Langton penned on April 8, 1841, in which she wrote:

> *We have been more fortunate with our poultry than any one of our neighbours. At the Falls weasels have been most destructive. We have seen none here except one, a beautiful white one, which I hope has left no progeny. This winter we have fed our poultry on grain. It may be rather expensive keep, but we had eggs during the winter and now abundance of them.*[69]

Exotic chickens, brought from Europe on merchant ships, became immensely popular among the wealthy or those aspiring to the upper class. The first poultry show was held in Boston in 1849, and the popularity of breeding fancy poultry rapidly spread to Canada. Having a clutch of showy chickens, though a status symbol, was also remarkably practical for a variety of reasons, not the least of which was diversity in the gene pool, a benefit that couldn't have been anticipated at the time.

CANADIAN TOMATO CHUTNEE.
A Testimonial received from
SIR JOHN A MACDONALD
PREMIER OF CANADA
I have tried your
TOMATO CHUTNEE
and found it very good.
yours very truly.
JOHN A MACDONALD
TEMPLUM FACIO
TRADE MARK.
TOMATO CHUTNEE.
FOR ROAST MEATS, STEAKS, CUTLETS, CURRIES, GRAVIES, GAME & SOUP.
POSSESSING A PIQUANCY OF FLAVOR AND FROM THE SUPERIORITY OF ITS
ZEST, IS MORE GENERALLY USED THAN ANY OTHER CONDIMENT.
PREPARED BY, M.P.C. GUELPH, ONTARIO CANADA.
REGISTERED.

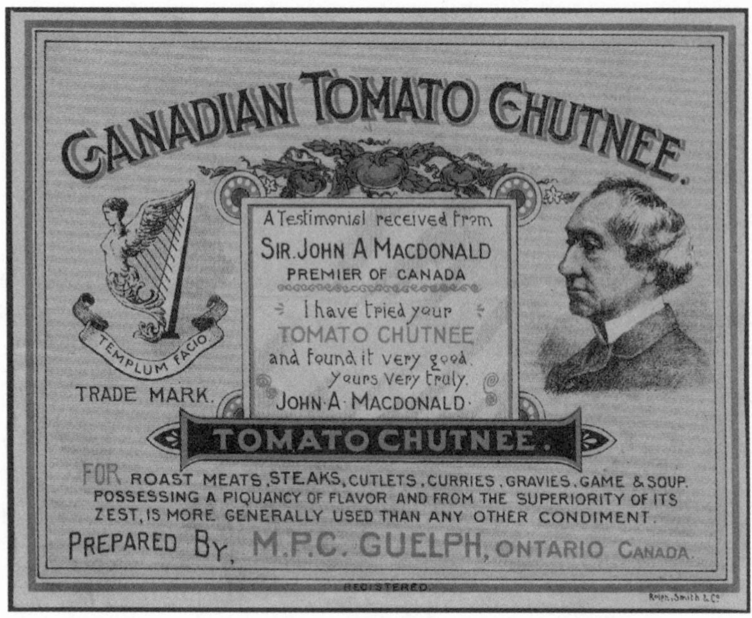

Sir John A. Macdonald apparently enjoyed Tomato Chutnee*

In her book on being a settler in Canada in mid-century, Catharine Parr Traill wrote: "In these days when all the world is running after Cochin China and Shanghai, Bantams and Dorkings, Dutch, Spanish, and Poland fowls, the omission of a chapter on the poultry-yard would, I fear, be regarded as a grave neglect in a work that is chiefly devoted to instruction on points of rural economy."[70]

Chickens were an important commodity to the settlers not just for eggs and meat, but also for cockfighting. Biographer P.B. Waite includes an excerpt about a cockfight west of Toronto in 1869 in his charming book *Macdonald: His Life and World.*

> [T]hey were a motley crew. For the most part they were rowdies of the purest breed — Toronto, London, Buffalo and Detroit were all represented by as scoundrelly a looking gang as it was possible to produce anywhere.... "Five — ten — fifteen — twenty dollars that the London bird wins," shouted a miserable ragamuffin who did not look as if he was worth five cents. "Make it a hundred and I take you," was the reply of a highly adorned young gentleman. "Done," said the ragamuffin, and he pulled from the pocket of his ragged trousers a bundle of bills amounting to several hundred and the bet was made. "Twenty-five cents on the Toronto bird, cried a miserable looking little old man; but the idea was altogether so low that down came a hand on the crown of his hat, and he was instantly extinguished.[71]

Early cookbooks contain a wide selection of recipes for chicken. Roast, baked, broiled, fried, fricasseed, jellied, curried, and served in a pie, chicken was a popular standby.

Curried dishes were surprisingly popular, having been incorporated into English cuisine from Asia. The British used the term *curry* to refer to both the collection of spices that make up curry powder and also to spicy dishes in general. An August 1839 entry in Anne Langton's diary shows that curry powder was available in Upper Canada: "Pickling has also been the order of the day. We consume more in the way of ketchups, sauces, curry powder, etc. than we used to at home, on account of the many months we are without fresh meat."[72]

---

* Judging by the picture of John A., this advertisement would likely have appeared in the 1880s. The portrait appears to be based on a photograph taken by William James Topley in 1883.

Chutney, also originating in South Asia, was a popular condiment served with cold meat or alongside a curry. John A. Macdonald liked chutney so much that he was prepared to have his face appear on a commercial endorsement.

The Canadian Home Cook Book, published in 1877 and "Compiled by Ladies of Toronto and Chief Cities and Towns in Canada," includes recipes for "Dal, An Indian Lentil," Bengal soup, curried chicken, "Curried Dishes," and just plain "Curry," as well as several types of pickles involving curry powder, cayenne, and turmeric, including India Pickle and East India Pickles.

The "Bengal Recipe for Making Mango Chetney," complete with spelling mistakes and Mrs. Beeton's comments, is from *Mrs. Beeton's Book of Household Management*, 1861.

CURRY. [submitted by] MISS BROKOVSKI

To make curry with rabbit, chicken, or any other meat, flour the meat and fry it a nice light brown; fry also two onions in the same way; mix a tablespoon of curry powder, and a small quantity of cayenne in a tea cup, with warm water to the consistency of cream and cover every part of the meat with the mixture; have ready some nice stock or thin gravy; put all together into a stew-pan and let it stew gently for twenty minutes; before serving slice two or three apples, let them stew away; this addition is thought to be a great improvement, as it makes the curry milder; rice to be boiled very dry and served around the dish.

BENGAL RECIPE FOR MAKING MANGO CHETNEY.

392. INGREDIENTS.—1-1/2 lbs. of moist sugar, 3/4 lb. of salt, 1/4 lb. of garlic, ¼ lb. of onions, 3/4 lb. of powdered ginger, 1/4 lb. of dried chilies, 3/4 lb. of mustard seed, 3/4 lb. of stoned raisins, 2 bottles of best vinegar, 30 large unripe sour apples.

Mode.— The sugar must be made into syrup; the garlic, onions, and ginger be finely pounded in a mortar; the mustard-seed be washed in cold vinegar, and dried in the sun; the apples be peeled, cored, and sliced, and boiled in a bottle and a half of the vinegar. When all this is done, and the apples are quite cold, put them into a large pan, and gradually mix the whole of the rest of the ingredients, including the remaining half-bottle of vinegar. It must be well stirred until the whole is thoroughly blended, and then put into bottles for use. Tie a piece of wet bladder over the mouths of the bottles, after they are well corked. This chetney is very superior to any which can be bought, and one trial will prove it to be delicious.

Note.—This recipe was given by a native to an English lady, who had long been a resident in India, and who, since her return to her native country, has become quite celebrated amongst her friends for the excellence of this Eastern relish.

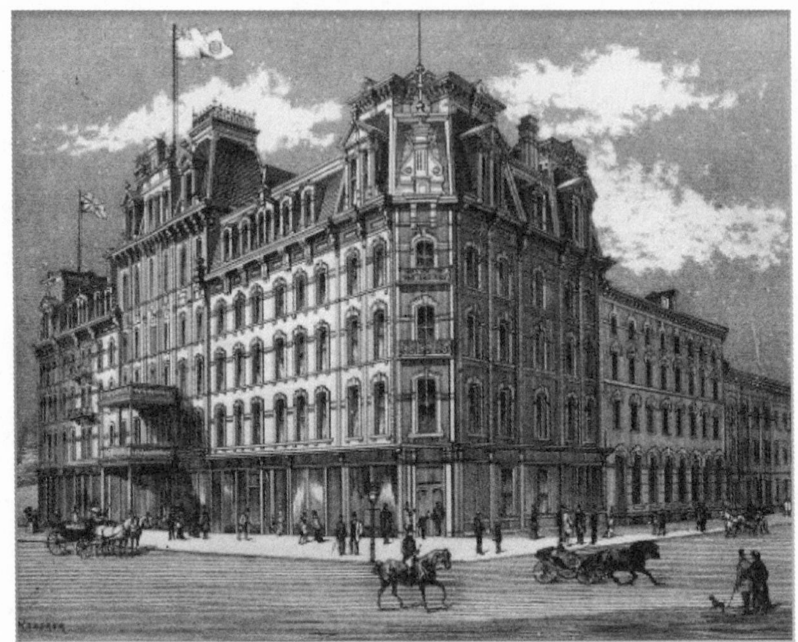

Russell House, circa 1893, by William James Topley

CHAPTER NINETEEN

The Phoenix Rises and Rewards a Thankful Nation

1873–79

If Macdonald felt disgraced over the Pacific scandal and his subsequent resignation, he certainly did not let it show, nor did he retreat. He continued daily life with his usual jauntiness, cockiness, and charm. On November 6, 1873, the day after his resignation as prime minister, he withdrew as Conservative Party leader, only to be promptly reinstated. A week after this, he attended a banquet held in his honour at the Russell House Hotel* and he was marched through the streets of Ottawa while a band played "When Johnny comes marching home again."

In the spring of 1874, fifty-nine-year-old Macdonald tried to resign again. He walked into the office of the Ottawa *Citizen* and asked that the newspaper announce his resignation from the Conservative Party. It declined. Their refusal signalled to Macdonald that he should stay on as a member of Parliament and as leader of the opposition.

---

* John A. was a regular at the Russell House, Ottawa's leading hotel prior to the building of the Chateau Laurier in 1912. Built in the 1840s, the Russell House was extensively renovated in the 1870s and 1880s. The hotel's prime location at the corner of Sparks Street and Elgin made it popular with politicians and visitors to Ottawa. In the late 1800s, a champagne lunch for two at the Russell House cost about three dollars, no tipping required. Accommodation and three meals ran between three and four dollars a night.

As usual, Macdonald was busy trying to raise much needed personal capital. He had moved his law firm from Kingston to Toronto in 1871 in order to be closer to the office of his main client, the Trust and Loan Company, and now he found himself shuttling between Ottawa and Toronto, where he was scrambling to resurrect his business. In 1875, he moved Agnes and Mary to a house on Sherbourne Street in Toronto.

Hugh John had been working in his father's law office, but this ended with an unfortunate family disagreement over his engagement to Jean King, a widow six years his senior, and worse than that, from John A.'s point of view, a Roman Catholic. When Hugh John wrote saying he was grieved that they should part in any disagreement and that he felt his father was acting "in an unnecessarily harsh manner" regarding his engagement, he signed off "Your obstinate but affectionate son, Hugh J. Macdonald." John A. accepted Hugh John's resignation without any argument, the same day he received it. His curt, formal answer was signed, "Yours truly, John A. Macdonald."

Hugh and Jean were married in Kingston where Hugh set up a law office on King Street, close to where his father had once practised law. John A. refused to attend the wedding, but the young couple were not rejected by Hugh's surrogate parents, James and Margaret Williamson.

Seeing Hugh John married was the last highlight of Margaret Macdonald Williamson's life. Hugh reported that she was extremely unwell, prompting John A. to write to Margaret's husband, James Williamson.

Ottawa Mar. 11, 1876

My dear Professor,

I need not tell you of my sorrow in the sad state of my dearest Sister.

She is my oldest and sincerest friend and has been so through life. I feel deeply for you. If I could be of any use I would at once go up and be with her. Let me know if you think I can. Hugh keeps me regularly informed of the state of matters. His letters allow no ground for hope.

Yours always
John A. Macdonald[73]

John A. never saw his sister again. She died shortly after the letter was sent. Normally this would have been an occasion for John A. to descend into an alcohol-induced haze. In the decade preceding, Macdonald's problem with alcohol had become much more pronounced. Always a binge drinker, the periods of inebriation had become more frequent, longer lasting, and alarming. There were stories of him staggering away from Parliament Hill so drunk that passersby gave him a wide berth. At one point during this era, Agnes walked out of a dinner leaving a very drunk and abusive John A. hurling insults at his hosts. But by the mid-1870s, Macdonald had more or less pulled himself together and beaten the worst of his addiction.

On the political front, Prime Minister Alexander Mackenzie had dealt with one problem after another. To begin with, Ontario was unhappy with the terms by which British Columbia joined the union. British Columbia's debts, coupled with the proposed costs of building the railway, made many in the East wonder if the financial burden would break the entire dominion. Since fifty of Mackenzie's seats were in Ontario, trying to keep these voters happy was a necessity. But British Columbia was not about to let the dominion off the hook. It had joined the union because of the promises made to it and threatened to secede if the pledged railway failed to materialize.

To compound matters, the world was in the midst of a massive depression, and as a result customs duties owed to Canada dried up. All over Europe and North America, factories were closing. In the Dominion of Canada, the Liberal government was committed to its stand against protection, arguing that protection would make things worse.

In 1876, the Tories adopted protection as part of their platform. In fact, being pro-protection might have been the single biggest factor in turning the Conservative fortunes around. John A. and Charles Tupper drafted a new national policy which would see duties lowered on necessities and raised on luxuries. Along with their protectionist platform they included pro-immigration and pro-railway policies. And then they took their show on the road.

From 1876 right through to 1878, the Conservative Party hosted a series of lively political picnics in Ontario and English-speaking Quebec. The picnics were a down-home, folksy, and hospitable way of getting the message to the people. It was a technique the Conservatives had mastered previously, and they resorted to it throughout the remainder of John A.'s career. The party provided large amounts of food and whisky while also paying lip service to the temperance movement. The food consisted of great hams, cold meat platters, roast turkeys, fried chicken, corn on the cob, homemade bread and buns, butter and cheese, devilled eggs, pickles and chutney, pound cakes, biscuits and preserves, along with lemonade and tea, and candies for the children. Macdonald's old friend Eliza Grimason played a role delivering food, kegs of whisky, and often John A. himself in her fine horse and buggy.

Hundreds turned out at every stop to hear Macdonald, the conjurer who had resurrected himself from political death and was now touting the merits of protection, something he had once argued against. It was not unusual for five hundred people or more to attend. Everywhere John A. went he charmed audiences as he always had. He bantered with the men drinking whisky. He stopped to talk to the women and ask their thoughts on political matters. He joked with the children. He was always at his best surrounded by people because he genuinely liked them. Few people could work a crowd like John A. He made everyone feel better. He was peddling hope in the midst of a depression.

On September 18, 1878, in the first election in Canada to use secret ballots rather than shouting out electoral choices, Macdonald was swept back into power in a Conservative majority, taking 134 of the 197 seats. There was just one predicament for Macdonald: he had lost in his own riding of Kingston, where voters felt that he deserted them when he moved his office and family to Toronto. Poor Eliza Grimason took the loss in Kingston hard. She told her beloved John A., "I went around town the next day cryin' til I hadn't an eye in my head."[74] Macdonald was elected soon after in a by-election in Victoria, British Columbia, although he had never been within two thousand miles of the city.

Macdonald had not only resurrected his political career and the fortunes of the Conservative Party, but he also managed to stay mostly sober. His addiction to alcohol, it seems, was only outweighed by his addiction to power and politics. Somehow, electioneering always brought out the best in John A. During the campaign, he repaired his relationship with Hugh John, whom he invited to return to the Toronto law office to take it over. Upon hearing this news, Patton, John A.'s partner in the firm, promptly resigned, giving John A. the opportunity to rename the firm Macdonald & Macdonald.

Perhaps John A.'s stance was softened when he learned the news of the birth of his first grandchild, baby Isabella, whom the family nicknamed Daisy. It was clear that John A. and Agnes were not likely to move back to Toronto any time soon, so they turned the lease of their Toronto home over to Hugh and his family. Sadly, Hugh John's wife, Jean, died shortly after due to complications from childbirth.

On October 17, 1878, Sir John A. Macdonald was sworn in as Canada's third prime minister. He and Agnes moved into Stadacona Hall on Laurier Avenue East, a grand home with space for family and entertaining. Mary was now nine years old. She was confined to a wheelchair, but she could speak slowly and read a little.

For the moment, at least, it was a golden time for John A., and for the nation. Macdonald's family were happy. The global depression was easing. The prospect of a transcontinental railway looked promising, and the plans were not yet obscured by the harsh realities of what it would take to build it.

Canada was soon to be home of a new governor general, the Marquess of Lorne and his wife, Princess Louise, daughter of Queen Victoria. The couple arrived in a snowstorm, on February 13, 1879, and went straight to Parliament Hill, where Lord Lorne opened the new session of Parliament. A week later, the couple hosted a state ball at Rideau Hall. Princess Louise, an avid cook who often made her own oyster pâté, even for major events, helped plan menus alongside the chef and kitchen staff.

Before the evening was out, John A. was once again drunk and, worse yet, either he or one of the senators—or perhaps both—had insulted Princess Louise by being overly familiar, possibly touching her and commenting on her figure. Like her mother, Princess Louise was not amused. Some sort of standoff prevailed.

A year later, Princess Louise returned to England. Most of John A.'s many biographers have assumed that she had had enough of Canada, but in fact, having suffered an accident, she sought to recuperate in her ancestral home, and it seems more than likely that she had had enough of Lord Lorne. Lorne had interests outside of marriage. A recent book about Princess Louise reveals that he was a rather flamboyant homosexual who frequently ventured out of the closet.[75]

Princess Louise was not a prude, although she was often portrayed that way. She was interested in women's rights. There were rumours she had male lovers—several of them. While in Canada, Louise took a lively interest in outdoor sports and in the First Nations. In the end, Louise parted friends with Macdonald and stayed in touch with him long after she returned to Britain. Lord Lorne remained in Canada for the duration of his tenure, and among other things, he grew fond of skating and tobogganing and travelled extensively throughout Canada.

If John A. suffered any guilt or embarrassment over that first diplomatic incident and breach of royal protocol, no one was any the wiser. It was well known that Macdonald despised pomposity in any form. He continued with business as usual, governing the country, enforcing protectionism, and building a railway. But first and foremost, before any of the other business was attended to, there was a new national holiday to be decreed. Commencing November 6, 1879, Parliament proclaimed that Canadians across the dominion would celebrate "a day of General Thanksgiving to Almighty God for the bountiful harvest with which Canada has been blessed."

THE FIRST OFFICIAL THANKSGIVING

The first Thanksgiving in Canada dates back to 1578 when English explorer Martin Frobisher was on his third trip to the Arctic searching for the Northwest Passage. Storms and calamities plagued the expedition, and the fleet of ships were separated. When they met again in what is now known as Frobisher Bay, expedition minister, Robert Wolfall, administered communion and delivered a sermon on thankfulness. Thus, Canadian Thanksgiving customs draw upon the Frobisher expedition's early prayers of gratitude, as well as on European peasants' harvest celebrations and American Pilgrim traditions.

The first official Thanksgiving dinners would have been surprisingly similar to many held in Canadian households today. Roast turkey and stuffing with gravy, a variety of cooked vegetables, and pumpkin, cranberry, and apple pies were all on the menu, even in 1879.

Much had changed since the Macdonald family first arrived in Canada West almost six decades earlier, when Helen Macdonald cooked dinners over the open hearth fire in pots hung over the coals. By the second half of the 1800s, although cooking was still an all-consuming effort, it was evolving. The first cooking stove was manufactured in the 1830s, near Long Point, Upper Canada by Joseph Van Nostrand. The stove stood only two feet tall, with four circular openings on top and a bake oven below. Slow to gain acceptance, by the late 1870s cast-iron cooking stoves, often heated with wood, were becoming more commonplace in Canadian homes. By the end of the nineteenth century, gas lighting and running water were available, but only to the wealthy households that had the means to enjoy such luxuries. By 1890 all the provinces had established electrical generating facilities and were working on distribution. In 1910, well after John A.'s lifetime, Berlin, Ontario (now Kitchener) became the first city in the nation to connect to a power grid. After World War I, with mass production, it became more commonplace for urban Canadian homes to have indoor plumbing and lighting.

The pace of the Columbian exchange—that is, the transfer of people, plants, animals, and diseases between the New World and the Old World, which is thought to have begun with Christopher Columbus—accelerated dramatically throughout the 1800s as the migration of goods and people across the Atlantic increased. New grocery products began to make significant transformations in the culinary palette. Some of these included baking powder and compressed yeast, powdered gelatin, refined sugar and flour, commercial ketchup and mustard, and baking chocolate, unsweetened, in disc form. In addition, Mason jars, invented and patented in 1858 by Philadelphia tinsmith John Landis Mason, revolutionized the preservation of fruit and vegetables, which had a positive impact on the availability of nutritious food, especially in winter.

There began a convergence of British, French, and First Nations food as corn, cranberries, pumpkin, blueberries, wild game, maple syrup, and, to a lesser extent, wild rice—all indigenous to North America—became standard fare in the Canadian diet.

By 1879, there was much to be thankful for in most Canadian kitchens, not the least of which was the new national holiday. Cranberry pie, sometimes called mock cherry pie, was one dish likely to be found on a many a Thanksgiving table. The pie made its first public appearance in *The Cook*

Not Mad and showed up again in later cookbooks, including *The Canadian Home Cook Book*. Both versions are included here. Imagination must be used to decipher the rather charming but cryptic instructions, especially from *The Cook Not Mad* recipes.

CRANBERRY PIE. MRS. P.

(from *The Canadian Home Cook Book*)

Take Cranberries, pick and wash them in several waters, and put them in a dish with the juice of half a lemon, quarter pound of moist sugar or pounded loaf sugar, to a quart of Cranberries; cover it with puff paste or short crust, and bake it three-quarters of an hour. If short crust is used, draw it from the oven five minutes before it is done, and ice it; return it to the oven, and send it to the table cold.

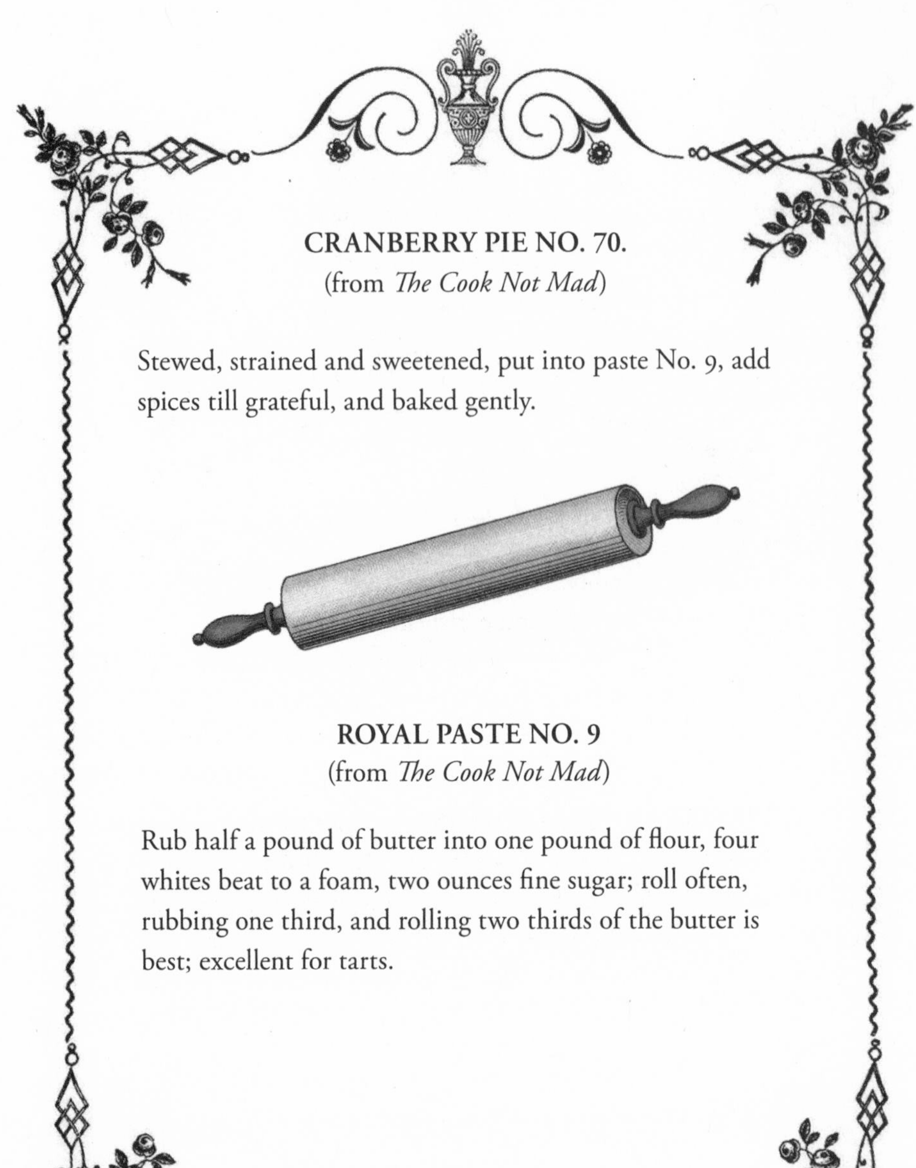

CRANBERRY PIE NO. 70.

(from *The Cook Not Mad*)

Stewed, strained and sweetened, put into paste No. 9, add spices till grateful, and baked gently.

ROYAL PASTE NO. 9

(from *The Cook Not Mad*)

Rub half a pound of butter into one pound of flour, four whites beat to a foam, two ounces fine sugar; roll often, rubbing one third, and rolling two thirds of the butter is best; excellent for tarts.

CHAPTER TWENTY

A Railway Runs through It

1880–86

At eight o'clock in the evening on Monday, June 28, 1886, the first Canadian transcontinental train left the station in Montreal bound for Port Moody, British Columbia, almost five thousand kilometres away. Five and a half days later, the train reached its final destination. This was now the longest railway line in the world, traversing the second largest country on Earth, through some of the most challenging and unforgiving geography on the planet. The improbable accomplishment of building a railway across Canada changed the nation forever. It provided a means of opening up the West and unifying the nation, and thus, advancing prosperity. But the building of it had taken a huge toll.

By 1880 Macdonald was assured that the Canadian Pacific Railway (CPR) syndicate would finance the railway and one year later the terms of the agreement with the government had been signed. From the beginning, this project was an epic and expensive headache, but Macdonald had staked his political career and the fortunes of the Conservative Party on it. He had made it into a symbol of the nation; failure was not an option.

The work was conducted simultaneously in three regions: Ontario, the Prairies, and British Columbia. In northern Ontario equipment sank into muskeg, while blackflies and mosquitos drove the workers mad. Granite had to be blasted through, swamps had to be filled, and lake levels had to be lowered. In the prairies, the land had to be cleared and then the foundation for the tracks secured. In the West, there was relentless danger. Precarious trestle bridges had to be built and tunnels blasted through rock. Cliffs and mountains had to be navigated, along with grizzly bears and cougars. The work was so dangerous, it is said that every mile of tunnel and track west of the prairies was stained with blood.

The forty thousand men who built the railway were called navvies. They were brought in from all over the world and paid around a dollar a day. They included Canadians, Americans, British, Irish, Italians, Swedish, and Chinese, who fared the worst. About fifteen thousand Chinese men were brought to the west coast in the hopes of escaping poverty and starvation at home, only to find a fate as bad, or worse, on the Canadian railroad. Many of them lacked appropriate attire and footwear. They had no warm clothing. They were fed starvation rations and did the most dangerous of all the jobs, often carrying huge weights and detonating dangerous, unstable explosives. They were paid less than half what the other workers earned and lived in appalling conditions as they tried to save money to send back to their families in China. There was no medical care for those who were injured or sick.

Many of the Chinese workers aspired to immigrate permanently and bring their families over. Their plans were thwarted when, in 1885, upon completion of the railway, the government introduced the Chinese Immigration Act, which forced all immigrants from China to pay a fifty dollar fee to enter Canada. Later, Prime Minister Wilfrid Laurier not only left the so-called Chinese head tax in place but raised the fee to $500. The tax remained in place until 1923.

The exploitation of railway workers by the Canadian government is one of the less popular chapters in the nation's history. They lived in deplorable conditions, were separated from their families, and were overworked and underpaid. If they complained, they were fired. An alarming number of the labourers fell ill from smallpox and cholera, and hundreds were killed or maimed in work-related accidents.

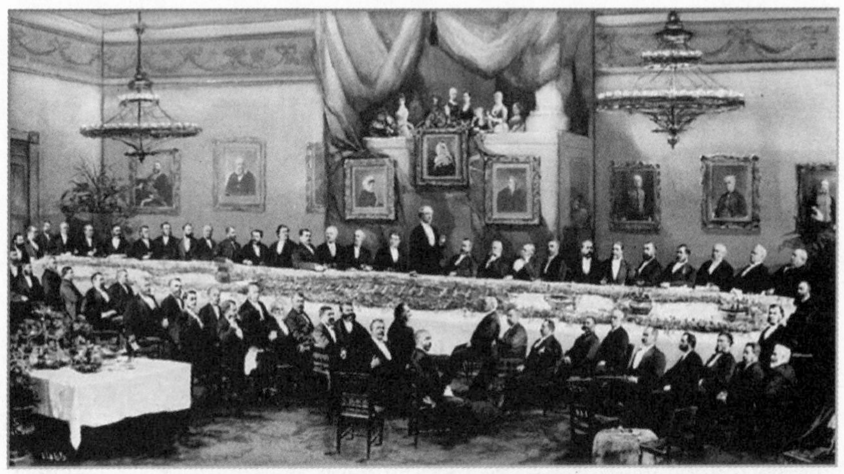

Old Guard Dinner by William James Topley, 1882

Early in 1882, partway through construction and before the full story was made public, Macdonald called an election. He was anxious to secure enough time at the helm in order to oversee the new national railway from start to finish.

On May 4, 1882, Macdonald attended a lavish Old Guard dinner held in his honour in the Commons Restaurant on Parliament Hill. The sixty guests included Sir John, Members of Parliament, Fathers of Confederation, and other important Canadians. William James Topley produced his famous composite photograph of the event by designing and painting the backdrop and then photographing each person after the event and pasting them onto the background. The composite was then photographed in its entirety and prints were sold.

In June, Macdonald was elected with his third majority government, and the nation immediately returned to the matter of the railway and settlement of the West. A program to provide wives for settlers in the prairies was abandoned by the Cabinet in 1882 on account of the number of "disreputable women" involved. John A. consoled a member of Parliament who was disheartened by the Cabinet's decision, telling him, "You know Angus, we must protect Canadian whores."[76]

By 1883, the CPR was in dire need of a fresh injection of money and had to ask the government for funds. Their request for $22.5 million was almost exactly equal to the entire federal revenue for the year. They were given the money as a loan, and from that point forward, the CPR teetered constantly on the edge of bankruptcy and came back again and again to the public coffer. Each time, the funds had to be approved by Parliament. By the time the railway was complete, it had cost the government $60 million in grants and $35 million in loans—almost $100 million, which was an astronomical amount of money at that time.

The great march west was marred by more than just the exploitation of workers both domestic and foreign—and staggering debts. It was also permanently damaged by the horrifying treatment of First Nations and the Métis people and the destruction of their traditional cultures and economies.

John A. Macdonald's "national dream" required clearing the land across the prairies in preparation for the laying of the track and settlement by Europeans. Thus began the collapse of the bison herds. The last hunt took place in 1879. For the indigenous people, bison were not just food. They used every part of the animal for sustenance, and for spiritual and material culture. Just as the bison disappeared, Lieutenant-Governor Edgar Dewdney cut rations and is purported to have sent to the Aboriginal people inferior, tainted food supplies, including pork that was unfit to eat and described as musty and rusty.[77] Under treaties signed with the First Nations, the government had promised not only food but also seeds and help with starting crops. But through a series of weather events and insect plagues, the crops failed and widespread malnutrition, famine, illness, and starvation ensued.

In the five years following the collapse of the bison herds, it is estimated that approximately three thousand indigenous people starved to death in the Northwest Territories,[78] a conservative number, since the area affected expanded beyond the Northwest Territories and deaths by disease were not included in the toll.

It was a horrifying and desperate situation exacerbated by lack of aid from the government, which was dealing with massive cost overruns on the CPR. Macdonald stands accused of starving the indigenous population in order to clear the plains, and while he was indeed prime minister, the Liberals in opposition complained that the government was spending too much on Indians, and turning them into permanent dependents.[79] In fact, the prevailing state of social consciousness at the time meant that Canadians stood by while disease and starvation decimated the First Nations people of the plains, along with the Métis.

When flooding rains deluged Saskatchewan in 1884, it was the final straw for the inhabitants. Frustrated by several years of bad luck and mistreatment, they sent for Louis Riel, who had become an American citizen and was living in Montana. Riel moved his family back to Canada and took stock of the situation. Unfortunately, Riel was mentally unstable and spent his time renaming the days of the week and the stars in the sky. He was, he said, a prophet and the pope of the New World. Nevertheless, he was able to gather together a force that would instigate rebellion.

In December 1884, the Métis nation sent a petition of grievances to Ottawa. One month later, the Cabinet authorized an investigation. Sensing that this was simply a delaying tactic, Riel and his men mounted a rebellion against the Dominion of Canada. On May 12, 1885, Riel gave himself up to the North West Mounted Police, and he was tried for high treason. Although his lawyer encouraged him to plead insanity, Riel refused as a point of honour. Public sentiment was running strongly against him because of the brutal murder of Thomas Scott in March 1870. On November 16, 1885, Riel was hanged in Regina at the North West Mounted Police quarters, along with eight other First Nations leaders.

This mass hanging and the handling of the settlement of the prairies remains one of the darkest periods in the history of Canada and a lasting black mark on the record of Sir John A. Macdonald, whose words and action were at odds. For example, he said, "The Indians are the aborigines — the original occupants of this country and their rights must be respected."[80]

In 1885, he proposed a bill giving First Nations the right to vote. This initiative was cancelled by Macdonald's successor, Wilfrid Laurier. Not until 1960 did Aboriginal people in Canada receive political franchise. Macdonald also wrote to Ojibwa Chief Dr. Peter Edmund Jones, saying that he wanted to see Indians placed on "a footing of equality with white brethren."[81] Dr. Jones, the first known Aboriginal person in Canada to graduate from medical school, received his degree in 1866, from Queen's College, Kingston. He was the son of Macdonald's close friend and trusted adviser, the Reverend Peter Jones (Kahkewaquonaby).

Elsewhere in the dominion, life went on. On December 18, 1884, Sir John A. Macdonald sat down with 1,200 guests for a spectacularly lavish dinner at the pavilion of the Horticultural Gardens in Toronto, at the launch of a new Liberal-Conservative Association for the Province of Ontario. John A. was unanimously elected as president of the association.

The banquet began with oyster soup, and progressed through several courses. Entrées included roast chicken, roast duck, roast goose, roast turkey, chicken mayonnaise, lobster salad, sugar-cured ham, tongue, partridge, and prairie chicken. For dessert there was lemon meringue pie, pound cake, almond macaroons, coconut kisses, port wine jelly, and a variety of fresh fruit, followed by a cheese course and, to bring it to completion, French coffee.

If anyone noticed the gross incongruity of the situation in light of what was happening on the plains, it wasn't mentioned. It is a telling fact that even the *Globe* missed the opportunity to take a stab at Sir John. In fact, the event was so popular that despite the 1,200 guests, there were many who were turned away and the galleries were filled with spectators, mainly women, who, it seemed, were content merely to view the grand banquet.

A year later, on November 2, 1885, just over two weeks before Riel was declared guilty, John A. and Agnes invited Justice Minister John Thompson to dinner. The Macdonalds were once again living at Earnscliffe, their old and much cherished home. It had come on the market in 1882, after owner Thomas Reynolds died, so the Macdonalds scraped together $10,000 for the purchase price and then spent almost as much again restoring and refurbishing the home.

Thompson recorded the particulars of that evening in a letter to his wife Annie, who was away and unable to attend.[82] When apart, the couple wrote to each other daily, and their informal and unreserved communication forms a wonderful source for day-to-day life in the late nineteenth century, full of many delightful details of the goings-on in Victorian Ottawa.

This was an elegant dinner. Thompson found the house beautiful, although perhaps in deference to his wife, he wrote that Lady Macdonald was very pleasant, "but as ugly as sin." Another guest, Lady Tilley, "tried to be very pleasant and did not need to try to be ugly." He also recorded the extravagant dinner menu, which would have been quite typical for a dinner party of the era, especially one hosted by the prime minister, even though it was just a Monday night.

The first course was oysters on the half-shell, which was followed by consommé, fish, lamb cutlets, and a variety of vegetables. For dessert there was cabinet pudding, charlotte russe, lemon ice, and fruit. It was usual to serve sherry before dinner and wine with the meal.

DESSERTS FIT FOR CABINET MINISTERS

Cabinet pudding and charlotte russe were popular puddings of the era. The first paid homage to Victorian England and the second, to France. Cabinet pudding may have seemed like an appropriate choice when entertaining cabinet ministers. It is a classic English steamed and moulded pudding, similar to bread pudding but made using sponge cake or jelly roll instead of stale bread. Recipes for cabinet pudding appeared in English, American, French, and Canadian cookbooks of the era with slight variations. It is also called chancellor's pudding or diplomat's pudding and, in France, it is known as pouding à la chancelière.

Charlotte russe is an elegant, light dessert made with sweetened, whipped cream, slightly set with gelatin and served inside a ring of savoy biscuits or ladyfingers. It was said to have been invented by the French chef Marie-Antoine Carême to honour both Princess Charlotte, daughter of his former employer, King George IV, and Carême's next employer, the Russian Czar Alexander I.

Gelatin became popular after 1845, when American industrialist, inventor, and candidate for the American presidency Peter Cooper successfully obtained a patent for powdered gelatin. Powdered gelatin replaced sheet gelatin, which required the time-consuming task of purification prior to use. Post 1845, charlotte russe was an extremely popular party dessert. The following recipe for cabinet pudding and this version of charlotte russe are from *Mrs. Beeton's Book of Household Management*.

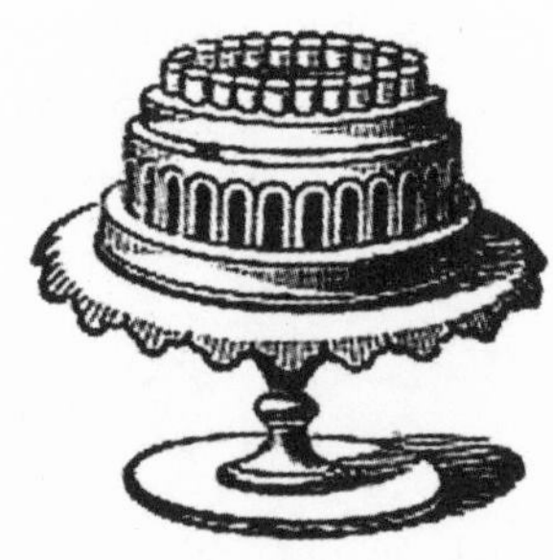

CABINET OR CHANCELLOR'S PUDDING

1256. INGREDIENTS.—1–1/2 oz. of candied peel, 4 oz. of currants, 4 dozen sultanas, a few slices of Savoy cake, sponge cake, a French roll, 4 eggs, 1 pint of milk, grated lemon-rind, 1/4 nutmeg, 3 table-spoonfuls of sugar.

Mode.—Melt some butter to a paste, and with it, well grease the mould or basin in which the pudding is to be boiled, taking care that it is buttered in every part. Cut the peel into thin slices, and place these in a fanciful device at the bottom of the mould, and fill in the spaces between with currants and sultanas; then add a few slices of sponge cake or French roll; drop a few drops of melted butter on these, and between each layer sprinkle a few currants. Proceed in this manner until the mould is nearly full; then flavour the milk with nutmeg and grated lemon-rind; add the sugar, and stir to this the eggs, which should be well beaten. Beat this mixture for a few minutes; then strain it into the mould, which should be quite full; tie a piece of buttered paper over it, and let it stand for 2 hours; then tie it down with a cloth, put it into boiling water, and let it boil slowly for 1 hour. In taking it up, let it stand for a minute or two before the cloth is removed; then quickly turn it out of the mould or basin, and serve with sweet sauce separately. The flavouring of this pudding may be varied by substituting for the lemon-rind essence of vanilla or bitter almonds; and it may be made much richer by using cream; but this is not at all necessary.

Time.—1 hour. Average cost, 1s. 3d.
Sufficient for 5 or 6 persons. Seasonable at any time.

CHARLOTTE RUSSE

1421. INGREDIENTS—About 18 Savoy biscuits, 3/4 pint of cream, flavouring of vanilla, liqueurs, or wine, 1 tablespoonful of pounded sugar, 1/2 oz. of isinglass [pure gelatin].

Mode.—Procure about 18 Savoy biscuits, or ladies'-fingers, as they are sometimes called; brush the edges of them with the white of an egg, and line the bottom of a plain round mould, placing them like a star or rosette. Stand them upright all round the edge; carefully put them so closely together that the white of the egg connects them firmly, and place this case in the oven for about 5 minutes, just to dry the egg. Whisk the cream to a stiff froth, with the sugar, flavouring, and melted isinglass [gelatin]; fill the charlotte with it, cover with a slice of sponge-cake cut in the shape of the mould; place it in ice, where let it remain till ready for table; then turn it on a dish, remove the mould, and serve. 1 tablespoonful of liqueur of any kind, or 4 tablespoonfuls of wine, would nicely flavour the above proportion of cream. For arranging the biscuits in the mould, cut them to the shape required, so that they fit in nicely, and level them with the mould at the top, that, when turned out, there may be something firm to rest upon. Great care and attention is required in the turning out of this dish, that the cream does not burst the case; and the edges of the biscuits must have the smallest quantity of egg brushed over them, or it would stick to the mould, and so prevent the charlotte from coming away properly.

Time.—5 minutes in the oven.
Average cost, with cream at 1s. per pint, 2s.
Sufficient for 1 charlotte. Seasonable at any time.

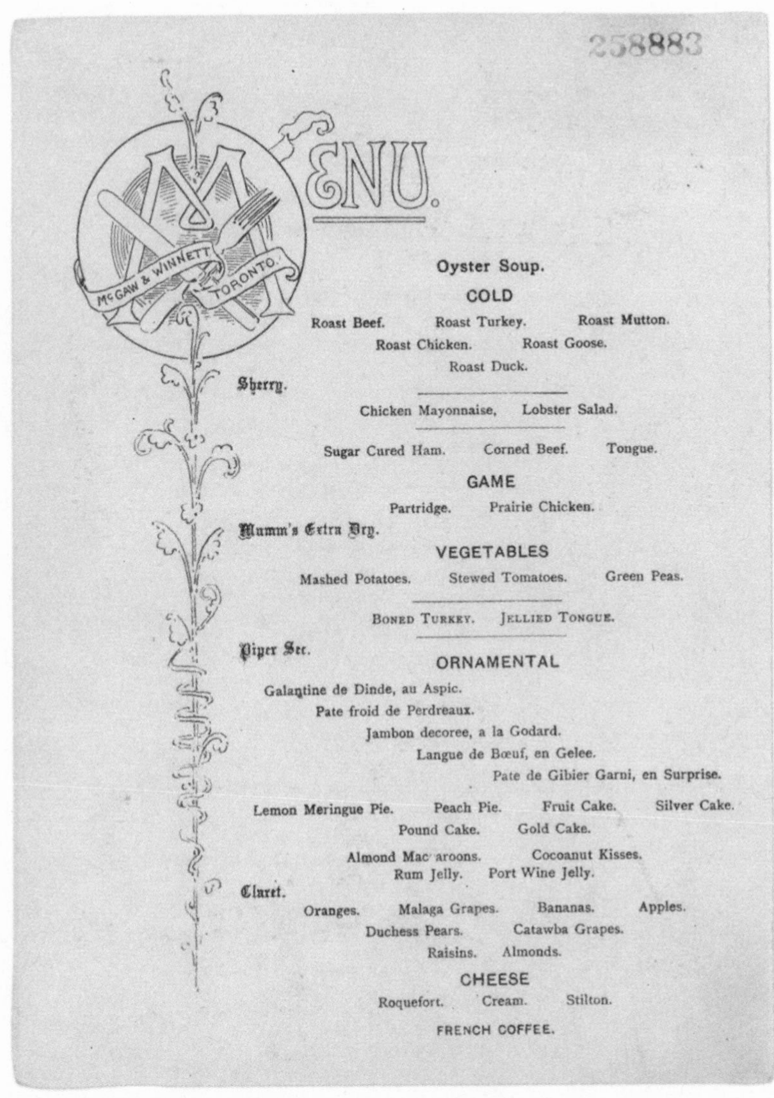

McGAW & WINNETT TORONTO.

MENU.

Oyster Soup.

COLD

Roast Beef. Roast Turkey. Roast Mutton.
Roast Chicken. Roast Goose.
Roast Duck.

Sherry.

Chicken Mayonnaise, Lobster Salad.

Sugar Cured Ham. Corned Beef. Tongue.

GAME

Partridge. Prairie Chicken.

Mumm's Extra Dry.

VEGETABLES

Mashed Potatoes. Stewed Tomatoes. Green Peas.

BONED TURKEY. JELLIED TONGUE.

Piper Sec.

ORNAMENTAL

Galantine de Dinde, au Aspic.
Pate froid de Perdreaux.
Jambon decoree, a la Godard.
Langue de Bœuf, en Gelee.
Pate de Gibier Garni, en Surprise.

Lemon Meringue Pie. Peach Pie. Fruit Cake. Silver Cake.
Pound Cake. Gold Cake.

Almond Macaroons. Cocoanut Kisses.
Rum Jelly. Port Wine Jelly.

Claret.

Oranges. Malaga Grapes. Bananas. Apples.
Duchess Pears. Catawba Grapes.
Raisins. Almonds.

CHEESE

Roquefort. Cream. Stilton.

FRENCH COFFEE.

Above and overleaf: Inside pages of menu and toasts booklet for banquet in honour of Sir John A. Macdonald, held on December 18, 1884

TOASTS.

1. THE QUEEN,
By the Chairman.

2. THE GOVERNOR-GENERAL AND LIEUTENANT-GOVERNOR,
By the Chairman.

3. THE ARMY, NAVY AND VOLUNTEERS,
By the Chairman.
To be responded to by the Hon. A. P. Caron, Minister of Militia.

4. OUR GUEST,
By the Chairman.

5. THE MINISTRY,
By Vice-Chairman of Table E.
To be responded to by Sir Hector Langevin and Sir David Macpherson.

6. THE SENATE,
By Vice-Chairman of Table F.
To be responded to by Sir Alex. Campbell.

7. THE HOUSE OF COMMONS,
By Vice-Chairman of Table D.
To be responded to by the Hon. J. A. Chapleau, Thos. White, M.P., and D'Alton McCarthy, Q.C., M.P.

8. THE LEGISLATIVE ASSEMBLIES OF THE PROVINCES,
By Vice-Chairman of Table G.
To be responded to by the Hon. Alex. Morris, M.PP. and the Hon. John Norquay.

9. OUR AGRICULTURAL INTERESTS,
By Vice-Chairman of Table H.
To be responded to by J. C. Rykert, M.P.

10. OUR MANUFACTURING INDUSTRIES,
By Vice-Chairman of Table C.
To be responded to by Thomas Cowan, Esq.

11. TRADE AND COMMERCE,
By Vice-Chairman of Table B.
To be responded to by Robert Henry, Esq.

12. THE LADIES,
By Vice-Chairman of Table A.

13. THE PRESS,
By the Chairman.

CHAPTER TWENTY-ONE

The End of the Line

1886–91

On July 10, 1886, John A. and Agnes climbed aboard the CPR train bound for the West. Their party of seven people were travelling in the luxurious Jamaica, a carriage named for Agnes's childhood home. The Jamaica was dark and sumptuous, upholstered with velvet and panelled with black walnut and cherry inlaid with brass. The bathrooms had ornate mirrors and marble basins and a claw-foot tub. The carriage windows were covered in wire mesh to keep out flies, sparks, and cinder. Railway screens were an innovation brought into the market in 1868, when an American patent had been filed for screened rail-car windows.

This was John A.'s first trip west. His previous travels had taken him only as far as west as Georgian Bay, Ontario. This fifty-day, six-thousand-mile round trip across the nation was to be a holiday of sorts that included inspection of the CPR and the beginning of the campaign for the upcoming 1887 election. There were whistle stops, photo ops, layovers, and various visits along the route. Macdonald and his party stopped in Winnipeg and disembarked from the train to meet Tory supporters. Amidst the cheering, Macdonald overheard one member of the crowd describe him as a seedy-looking old beggar. Macdonald didn't miss a beat, shooting back, "Yes, a rum 'un to look at, but a rare 'un to go."[83] On another occasion he told the assembled audience that he was surprised that the building of the railway had not killed him and that his friends thought he might see the final version from heaven, while his enemies expected he'd have to look up from below. "I've now disappointed both friends and foes," he quipped cheerfully, "and am taking the horizontal view."[84]

In Regina, John A.'s party was joined by Lieutenant-Governor Edgar Dewdney, who was also Indian commissioner for the Northwest Territories. They were scheduled to meet with Chief Crowfoot of the Blackfoot Tribe, in Gleichen, east of Calgary, in what was later to become the province of Alberta.

Joseph Pope, John A.'s private secretary, recorded this impression of the landscape:

> Imagine a boundless plain, perfectly level, covered with short wavy grass, not a tree or a bush of any kind.... The buffalo had disappeared some years before, but every now and then one could perceive their bones bleaching on the prairie.... In 1882 there were 100,000 skins sold in St. Paul, and in 1883 just four.[85]

Agnes, who was also busy writing a travelogue entitled "By Car and By Cowcatcher" for the monthly *Murray's Magazine* in London, England, wrote of the "soft, rapid tread of many moccasined feet" passing near their car as the people assembled. Chief Crowfoot explained to Macdonald that his people had been happy with plenty of food until white men had come and taken their land, killed off their buffalo, and deprived them of their means to live. A translator hired to interpret Crowfoot's speech to the dignitaries appears to have been woefully inadequate. The interpreter listened intently to Crowfoot's impassioned speech and when he stopped for breath, Lieutenant-Governor Dewdney turned to the interpreter, who shuffled his feet and said, "He says he damn glad to see you." Crowfoot resumed his lengthy speech

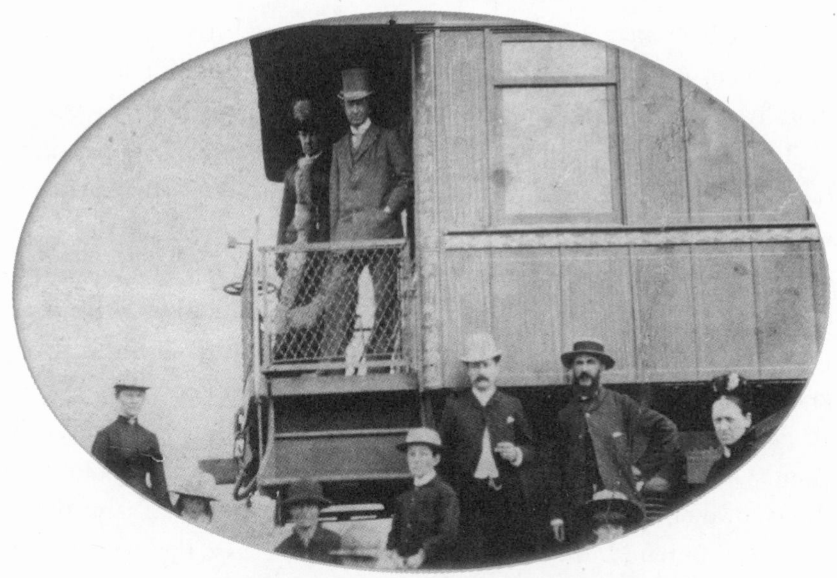

Sir John and Lady Macdonald at a whistle stop in Port Arthur, Ontario, September 3, 1886

making gestures to the sun, sky, and landscape. Again he paused, and the dignitaries turned to the interpreter, who after some hesitation managed to come up with, "He say he damn hungry."[86] At this, Crowfoot protested his loyalty, and Sir John invited all present to join in a banquet and offered gifts of pipes, tea, and tobacco.[87]

From Gleichen, the train headed into the mountains whereupon, much to everyone's amazement and concern, Agnes insisted on riding the cowcatcher — the pronged metal beak mounted to the front of the locomotive designed to remove obstacles, such as dead livestock, from the tracks in order to prevent the train from derailing. When she asked John A. if she might ride the cowcatcher, he was dismissive. "That's rather ridiculous," he told her.[88] Undeterred nonetheless, for the last six hundred miles of the trip, Agnes was atop her pillow, strapped to the cowcatcher, enjoying her rollercoaster ride. Egged on by Agnes, John A. agreed to join her briefly, but his tolerance was short-lived, and he soon returned the comfort of his chair in the caboose.

The train chugged to the top of the Continental Divide, 5,339 feet (1,627 metres) above sea level, before cutting off the steam and speeding down the western side of Kicking Horse Pass, a 4.5 percent gradient, the steepest and one of the most dangerous stretches of railroad in North America. In 1909, after several accidents, the CPR opened a pair of spiral tunnels to navigate the pass, which added several kilometres to the route but reduced the dangerous grade to a much more manageable 2.2 percent.

At 1 p.m. on Saturday, July 24, Macdonald's train pulled into Port Moody, British Columbia—the end of the line. At this triumphant moment for John A., a crowd of well-wishers came to witness his arrival, as a Pacific breeze blew in off Burrard Inlet. Macdonald had finally traversed the country along the railway that he dreamed would unite Canada.

Soon after, Macdonald and his party set off by steamboat for Victoria, the city that had elected him to Parliament in 1878, although he had never been there. They stayed for three weeks at the Driard House, said to be one of the best hotels on the continent, with a reputation for its outstanding food, as cited by Macdonald's biographer P.B. Waite:

> Fresh salmon, small coppery oysters . . . a few hours out of the sea, English pheasant, beautifully cooked splendid crabs, every known vegetable, a real master piece of a sweet . . . all washed down by the finest vintages that ever came "round the Horn," and then such cigars and such coffee![89]

By September, John A. was back in Ottawa, preparing for the next federal election. There were several dark clouds in the political skies. For example, the hanging of Louis Riel divided the nation with many feeling Macdonald should have shown leniency. In the Northwest, there was still tension from the rebellion of 1885. In Quebec, the Conservative Party was lacking support. The national policy was not producing expected results, and the country seemed once again to be heading towards economic depression. The financial fallout of the CPR was causing many to question its value. Of particular concern were the assaults being made by the four Liberal premiers of Nova Scotia, Manitoba, Quebec, and Ontario on the authority of the dominion government. In particular, Macdonald's former articling law student and long-time political adversary Oliver Mowat, now the premier of Ontario, seemed intent on making the province a sovereign state. When Macdonald was asked what he thought of his rival, he replied in characteristic fashion, "I have always been greatly impressed by his handwriting."[90]

Things did not look good for John A., and a new Liberal government for Canada seemed altogether possible. Nevertheless, against all advice to the contrary, Macdonald called the election for February 1887. He was running again in Kingston. Seventy-one-year-old Macdonald kept up an incredible pace throughout the campaign, travelling through blizzards, attending meeting after meeting, and making numerous speeches. The *Globe* referred to Macdonald as a tired old plough horse, prompting John A. to remind Canadians that the *Globe* had also once reported on his suicide. Although many people predicted a Liberal government, on February 22, 1887, Sir John won another majority government and was returned to his seat in Kingston.

There were rumours afoot that Macdonald was considering a journey to England, where he might be named to the House of Lords, or alternately, that he might be sent to Washington as an ambassador. Either of these was seen to be a fitting closure to a forty-five-year career in politics. During his years at the helm he had been instrumental in the establishment of confederation, he had overseen the building of a transcontinental railway, he had fought to protect Canada's rights and deftly handled relations with the United States of America, he had been instrumental in the established of the North West

Mounted Police, and he had sought to maintain French–English relations in Canada to keep a balance between their competing interests.

His wisdom in politics, his passion for Canada, his generosity, his wit, and his many accomplishments were legendary. Despite all this, John A. Macdonald simply could not afford to retire. With no pension and no significant savings outside of the trust fund that his friends and supporters had set up for his family, he needed to continue to make his salary, now $8,000 a year. This was his major motivation for continuing in politics, to provide for the family, especially for his daughter Mary, who was now eighteen years old. Although her mental acuity had surpassed all expectations, she would never work nor marry.

Macdonald's search for a successor was likely half-hearted. He had lived hard and worked hard for a very long time and was enjoying this period of grace in his life. He was healthier and looking better than he had for a long time. Agnes pronounced him "shiny." Fifteen-year-old Lucy Maud Montgomery met Macdonald in 1890 and called him "a spry-looking old man — not handsome but pleasant-faced." The same year a visitor to Sir John's office commented that he was still cracking jokes and that on receiving callers, he gave a skip and poked one of them in the ribs with his cane.[91]

When the Reverend Byron H. Stauffer gave an address to the Empire Club in Toronto in 1915, he remembered Macdonald, the Old Chieftain, in a surprisingly moving speech:

> He was born a leader; he had that peculiar quality which we call magnetism, which I suppose is another word for love. Magnetism is that quality which compels a man to walk ten blocks out of his way to meet you, instead of walking ten blocks out of his way to avoid you. Magnetism was the quality which Sir John held. A country member of Parliament — I think his name was David Thompson of Haldimand — said,

"I was sick nearly all the session, and at last I went back to Ottawa. The first man I met was Blake; he passed me with a simple nod as if he had forgotten I was away. Then I met Cartwright, who was just as cold. Then I met Sir John, who rushed across the chamber, slapped me on the shoulder, grasped my hand, and said, 'Davy, I am glad you are back again; I hope you will live many a day to vote against me.' It was pretty hard not to follow a man like that."

He had a great heart, as big a heart as ever beat within a human breast. He was always thoughtful of the feelings of the other fellow. He had an old lawyer named McIntosh in his office in Kingston, who was getting so old that he was absolutely useless, and yet he came down every morning and went through the motions; until one day, knowing that he could not earn his money, he went to John A. and said, "Mr. Macdonald, I will have to give up, I know I am useless to you." And he put his arm around the old lawyer and said, "Why, Mr. McIntosh, I couldn't open the office without you in the morning; you look after the law students, you see that they do their work right; you open the office; you get the newspapers ready for me, and show me the leading legal news in the morning. You must stay here, and if you insist on it I will just raise your wages a bit; I don't want any other lawyer in town to get you."[92]

Rev'd Stauffer's entire lengthy speech is peppered with similar anecdotes of Sir John's humility and compassion, of how he could take a disparate bunch of men and unite them, of how he referred to himself as a cabinet-maker, of his prodigious memory, and of his ability to shed tears.

He had a heart that was easily touched. When David Mills exonerated

Hugh John, Sir John's son, in connection with some corruption charges, the veteran premier, his eyes full of tears, crossed the House to thank his adversary. When Thomas White died, Sir John arose to speak, and after saying, "Mr. Speaker," sank to his chair, threw his head on his desk, and sobbed with unutterable sorrow.[93]

Macdonald ran one last time. The Liberals were running with a campaign of reciprocity with the United States that many, including the *Globe*, feared would lead to American annexation of Canada. Macdonald's campaign was based on loyalty—to the Dominion of Canada, to Britain, to his supporters, his family, and his friends. His good friend Sir Charles Tupper, who had returned to England, came back to Canada to be at John A.'s side. The CPR stood by Macdonald, too. On March 5, 1891, seventy-six-year-old Macdonald won his fifth and final term as prime minister.

In one of the happiest and most poignant moments of Sir John's life, his son Hugh John was elected as the member of Parliament for Winnipeg. Father and son took their oaths together, and then entered the House of Commons arm in arm.

By May, John A. was gravely ill. He suffered a stroke that left him lingering between life and death. He died on June 6, 1891 at his beloved Earnscliffe. Joseph Pope, Sir John A. Macdonald's private secretary, stood at the garden gates addressing the correspondents gathered there. "Gentleman," Pope said, "Sir John Macdonald is dead."

Pope then posted a notice on the gate which read:

Earnscliffe, 10.30 p.m.
Sir John Macdonald died at 10.15 p.m.
(signed) R.W. Powell, M.D.

An hour later the sign was stolen.

The following day the *Globe* ran the stark headline, "The Dead Premier."[94]

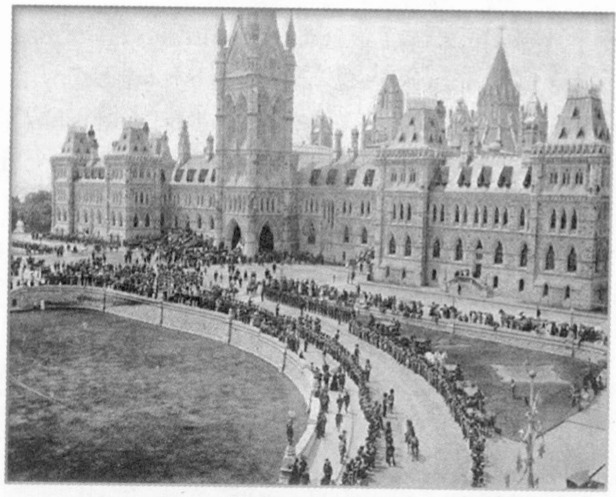

Sir John A. Macdonald's funeral procession
on Parliament Hill, Ottawa, June 1891

Wilfrid Laurier, the leader of the Liberal Party who went on to become the next prime minister, said in Parliament, "In fact the place of Sir John A. Macdonald in this country was so large and so absorbing that it is almost impossible to conceive that the politics of this country, the fate of this country, will continue without him. His loss overwhelms us."[95]

The nation mourned Macdonald's loss. He lay in state in an open casket in the Senate Chamber in Parliament with rare white roses sent from Queen Victoria on his chest. His casket was then moved by railway to Kingston, where he lay in state in Kingston's City Hall and was remembered by those who had knew him as family, friend, or neighbour. A memorial service was held at Westminster Abbey in England, attended by the Sovereign and her family. He was buried alongside his father Hugh, his mother Helen, his first wife Isabella and their infant son, John Alexander, and his sisters Margaret and Louisa. In the years to follow, his dear friend Eliza Grimason was buried in a plot adjacent to the Macdonald family.

The Great Chieftain, who had worked from the age of fifteen until the month of his death, had died in the harness, poor but happy, reunited with his son, surrounded by family and friends, and knowing that his mourners would continue to remember him, for better or worse, for decades and centuries to come.

Macdonald asked Canadians for forgiveness of his "sins of omission and commission," which he did not deny, and asked we remember instead that "in the ultimate issue... he loved much."[96]

A PUDDING IN HIS HONOUR

In honour of the Old Chieftain, there is a recipe in the 1888 publication *Dora's Cook Book*, which is called Sir John A. Pudding.

The only known publicly available copy of *Dora's Cook Book* in Canada is located in the Lennox and Addington Museum and Archives, in Napanee, Ontario, although other copies may exist in private collections. Dora E. Fairfield was twenty-six years old and single when her 311-page cookbook was published by Hunter, Rose, and Co., in 1888. She included recipes for all the standard fare of the day: roast goose, potted pigeon, curried chicken, cranberry sauce, watercress salad, scrambled eggs, scalloped frogs, cabbage salad, and burnt butter sauce for fish.

Dora listed cooking times for a long list of vegetables. She suggested thirty minutes for cooking potatoes and a rather astonishing one to two hours cooking time for carrots and green beans. Her recipe for salmon salad called for a can of salmon. Although cans had been in existence since 1813, they rarely cropped up in cookbooks during the 1800s. Dora also included an essay on how to boil an egg; a topic that many famous food writers have written about since. Her instructions begin with very contemporary sounding lines:

> Science shows that the best way to boil an egg is not to boil it; the old three minute rule is entirely out of date. Put the eggs in the saucepan when the water is boiling, the cold eggs will lower the temperature from 212 degrees [Fahrenheit] to less than 200 degrees; place the dish on the back of the stove where it will keep hot, and in ten minutes the eggs will be ready to serve.

Here, with its very incomplete instructions, is the pudding Dora Fairfield named for Sir John A. Macdonald.

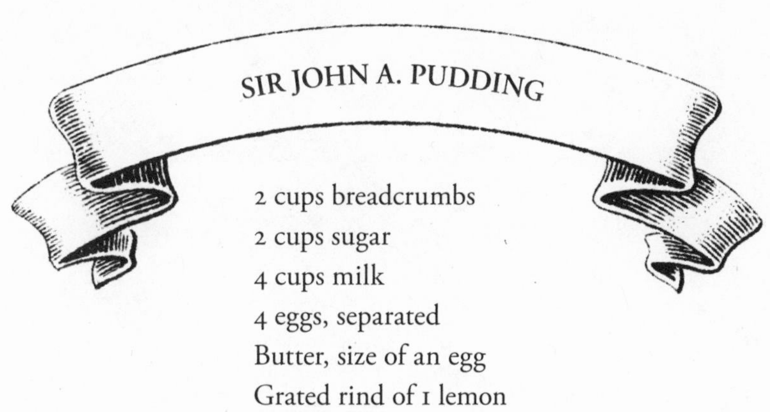

SIR JOHN A. PUDDING

2 cups breadcrumbs
2 cups sugar
4 cups milk
4 eggs, separated
Butter, size of an egg
Grated rind of 1 lemon

Beat the eggs yolks well. Combine with the breadcrumbs, milk, butter and lemon rind. Stiffly beat the egg whites. Sprinkle sugar over the top when done. Spread over the top of the pudding. Bake in oven a few minutes and serve with butter.

Notes

1 Emerson Bristol Biggar, *Anecdotal Life of Sir John Macdonald* (Montreal: Lovell, 1891), 28.

2 Catharine Parr Traill, *The Backwoods of Canada: Being Letters from the Wife of an Emigrant Officer, Illustrative of the Domestic Economy of British America* (London: C. Knight, 1836), 320.

3 Patricia Phenix, *Private Demons: The Tragic Personal Life of John A. Macdonald* (Toronto: McClelland & Stewart, 2006), 17.

4 Joseph Pope, *Memoirs of the Right Honourable Sir John Alexander Macdonald, G.C.B., First Prime Minister of the Dominion of Canada*, vol. 1 (Ottawa: J. Durie & Son, 1894), 6-7.

5 Ged Martin, *John A. Macdonald: Canada's First Prime Minister* (Toronto: Dundurn Press, 2013), 28.

6 Biggar, *Anecdotal Life of Sir John Macdonald,* 46.

7 Ibid., 47.

8 Phenix, *Private Demons*, 22.

9 Richard Gwyn, *John A: The Man Who Made Us* (Toronto: Random House, 2008), 31.

10 Ged Martin, "Sir John Eh? Macdonald: Recovering a Voice From History," *British Journal of Canadian Studies* 17, no. 1 (2004): 117-24.

11 Martin, *John A. Macdonald,* 32-33.

12 Pope, *Memoirs,* vol. 1, 11.

13 Keith Johnson, *Affectionately Yours: The Letters of Sir John A. Macdonald and His Family* (Toronto: Macmillan of Canada, 1969), 29.

14 Biggar, *Anecdotal Life,* 52.

15 Phenix, *Private Demons,* 58.

16 Lt. Col. J. Pennington Macpherson, *The Life of the Rt. Hon. Sir John A. Macdonald* (St. John, NB: Earle Publishing House, 1891), 4-5.

17 Johnson, *Affectionately Yours,* 32.

18 Ibid., 34-35.

19 Ibid., 35.

20 Ibid., 41.

21 Martin, *John A. Macdonald*, 50.

22 Johnson, *Affectionately Yours*, 58.

23 James McSherry, "The Invisible Lady: Sir John A. Macdonald's First Wife," *Canadian Bulletin of Medical History* 1, no. 1 (1984): 92-93, 96.

24 Phenix, *Private Demons,* 103.

25 Hugh Hornby Langton, ed., *A Gentlewoman in Upper Canada: The Journals, Letters and Art of Anne Langton* (Toronto: Clarke, Irwin, 1950), 189.

26 Johnson, *Affectionately Yours*, 72-73.

27 Gwyn, *John A,* 128.

28 Donald Swainson, *Sir John A. Macdonald: The Man and the Politician*, 2nd ed. (Kingston, ON: Quarry Press, 1989), 42.

29 Johnson, *Affectionately Yours,* 89.

30 Ibid., 91-92.

31 Martin, *John A. Macdonald,* 76.

32 Phenix, *Private Demons,* 135-36.

33 P.B. Waite, *Macdonald: His Life and World* (Toronto: McGraw-Hill Ryerson, 1975), 13.

34 Macpherson, *Life*, 425.

35 Swainson, *Sir John A. Macdonald,* 54.

36 Martin, *John A. Macdonald,* 79.

37 Johnson, *Affectionately Yours,* 96-97.

38 Swainson, *Sir John A. Macdonald,* 56.

39 P.B. Waite, *The Charlottetown Conference* (Ottawa: Canadian Historical Association, No. 15, 1970), 11.

40 Gwyn, *John A,* 304.

41 Ibid., 276.

42 Ged Martin, "John A. Macdonald and the Bottle," *Journal of Canadian Studies* 40, no. 3 (2006): 162-85.

43 Rev. Francis W.P. Bolger, "The Charlottetown Conference and Its Significance in Canadian History," *Canadian Catholic Historical Association*, report no. 27 (1960): 18.

44 Martin, *John A. Macdonald,* 89.

45 Johnson, *Affectionately Yours,* 98-99.

46 Gwyn, *John A*, 387.

47 Johnson, *Affectionately Yours,* 102-103.

48 Louise Reynolds, *Agnes: The Biography of Lady Macdonald* (Toronto: Samuel Stevens, 1979), 45.

49 Ibid.,51.

50 Phenix, *Private Demons,* 183.

51 Ibid., 184.

52 Reynolds, *Agnes,* 58.

53 Phenix, *Private Demons*, 196.

54 Reynolds, *Agnes,* 65.

55 Ibid., 58.

56 Martin, *John A. Macdonald,* 122.

57 Biggar, *Anecdotal Life of John A. Macdonald*, 233.

58 Steven Poole, "Queen Victoria on cannabis, and all the other things you never knew about drugs," *New Statesman*, February 14, 2014, http://www.newstatesman.com/2014/02/high-hopes.

59 Phenix, *Private Demons,* 212.

60 Waite, *Macdonald*, 51.

61 Phenix, *Private Demons,* 214.

62 Ibid., 215.

63 Richard Gwyn, *Nation Maker: Sir John A. Macdonald: His Life, Our Times* (Toronto: Vintage, 2012), 213.

64 Johnson, *Affectionately Yours,* 111-12.

65 Swainson, *Sir John A. Macdonald,* 98-99.

66 Macpherson, *Life*, 199.

67 Ibid.

68 Swainson, *Sir John A. Macdonald*, 99.

69 Langton, *A Gentlewoman in Upper Canada,* 321.

70 Catharine Parr Traill, *The Female Emigrant's Guide and Hints on Canadian Housekeeping* (Toronto: Maclear, 1854), 133-34.

71 Waite, *Macdonald,* 49-50.

72 Langton, *A Gentlewoman in Upper Canada,* 252.

73 Johnson, *Affectionately Yours,* 118.

74 Phenix, *Private Demons,* 245.

75 Lucinda Hawksley, *The Mystery of Princess Louise: Queen Victoria's Rebellious Daughter* (London: Random House, 2013), 181.

76 Waite, *Macdonald*, 50.

77 James William Daschuk, *Clearing the Plains: Disease, Politics of Starvation, and the Loss of Aboriginal Life* (Regina: University of Regina Press, 2013), 118.

78 Margaret Conrad and Alvin Finkel, *History of the Canadian Peoples, 1867 to the Present*, vol. 2, 4th ed. (Toronto: Pearson, 2005).

79 Richard Gwyn, "Canada's First Scapegoat," *The Walrus*, December 2014, http://thewalrus.ca/canadas-first-scapegoat/.

80 Martin, *John A. Macdonald*, 167.

81 Gwyn, *Nation Maker*, 420.

82 John Thompson to Annie Thompson, *Sir John Thompson Papers*, vol. 288, November 3, 1885. Library and Archives Canada.

83 Gwyn, *Nation Maker*, 9.

84 Patricia Beeson, *Macdonald Was Late For Dinner* (Peterborough, ON: Broadview Press, 1993), 191.

85 Reynolds, *Agnes*, 110.

86 Maurice Pope, ed., *Public Servant: The Memoirs of Sir Joseph Pope* (Toronto: Oxford University Press, 1960), 54-55.

87 Reynolds, *Agnes*, 111.

88 Phenix, *Private Demons*, 271.

89 Waite, *Macdonald*, 168.

90 Richard Gwyn, "Sir John A. Macdonald made mistakes, but he wasn't a racist," *Toronto Star*, February 6, 2014.

91 Martin, *John A. Macdonald*, 178.

92 Rev. Byron H. Stauffer, speaker, Address to The Empire Club of Canada, Toronto, February 18, 1915, http://speeches.empireclub.org/62057/.

93 Ibid.

94 *Globe and Mail*, http://v1.theglobeandmail.com/series/primeministers/stories/obit-JAM.html.

95 Swainson, *Sir John A. Macdonald*, 148.

96 Pope, *Memoirs*, vol. 2 (Ottawa: J. Durie & Son: Ottawa, 1894), 293.

Acknowledgements

First, to my family — Chris, Laura, and Elysia — thank you for your constant love and support.

My sincere gratitude to everyone at Goose Lane Editions and especially to Colleen Kitts for believing in this book with only forty pages of manuscript to work with; to Julie Scriver for vital artistic contributions; to Jill Ainsley for invaluable and much needed proofreading and fact checking; and to Martin Ainsley for your patience and expertise as production editor. It has been a privilege to work with all of you. Thank you to Elizabeth Eve for editing my manuscript.

Special thanks to Ken Cuthbertson, former editor of the *Queen's Alumni Review* and Don Gillmor, author of *Canada: A People's History*, for your vital roles in making this book happen.

Huge heartfelt gratitude to the *New Quarterly* for sponsoring me to attend the annual Write on the French River retreat at Pine Cove where I first worked on this manuscript.

David More for sharing your old Montreal family recipe for tourtière and Paul Fortier, owner of Sir John's Public House in Kingston, for the treasured historic shortbread recipe — thank you both.

To my friends and family for your support and encouragement — thank you all. And for your presence in my life while I was writing this book: thank you Joy McNevin, Karen Rudie, Joanne Karaiskakis, Liz Flynn, Linda Ann Daly, Jackie King, Bruce Kauffman, Kat Evans, Carole Dufort, and Jennifer Smeltzer.

My gratitude to all the talented writers who have helped me along my path, including Helen Humphreys, Diane Schoemperlen, Oakland Ross, Isabel Huggan, Elizabeth Greene, Laurie Gough, and especially to my mentor, Susan Scott, lead non-fiction editor at the *New Quarterly*.

To everyone at Wintergreen Studios Press — my sincere appreciation.

To Madeleine Trudeau, curator of the Sir John A. Macdonald collection, and staff at Library and Archives Canada; George Muggleton, Interpretation Officer at Bellevue House; Jane Foster and staff at the Lennox and Addington County Museum and

Archives; staff at Archives of Ontario; Canadian Pacific Railway Archives; and the staff at the Kingston Frontenac Public Library—heartfelt thanks for your assistance.

I owe a debt of gratitude to the many biographers and historians who researched and wrote about Sir John A. Macdonald before me and to Sir John himself, who once roamed the same streets I now roam.

Finally, my sincere thanks to the Ontario Arts Council for financial support at various times throughout the past few years.

Illustration Credits

6 Portrait of John A. Macdonald by William McFarlane Notman. City of Vancouver Archives, CVA 371-1699.

23 "A New Map of Upper and Lower Canada, 1798." Originally published by Stockdale Piccadilly. Samuel Peter Jarvis and William Dummer Powell Collection. Ref. code: F 31-B-36-03, Image no.: I0028705. Archives of Ontario.

30 "Hugh Macdonald's store in Kingston." From E.B. Biggar, *Anecdotal Life of Sir John Macdonald*, 1891. Courtesy of Toronto Public Library.

30 "The Macdonald homestead at Adolphustown." From E.B. Biggar, *Anecdotal Life of Sir John Macdonald*, 1891. Courtesy of Toronto Public Library.

36 "Helen Shaw Macdonald, ca. 1850." Daguerreotype, Library and Archives Canada, a134902.

50 "John A. Macdonald's receipt for application to the Law Society of Upper Canada." Library and Archives Canada, c90940.

51 "John A. Macdonald's stone house on Rideau Street, Kingston." Library and Archives Canada, c004508.

61 "Portrait of Isabella Clark" by William Sawyer. Library and Archives Canada, c098673k.

64 "Statement of Marriage between John A. Macdonald and Isabella Clark." Library and Archives Canada, e008303545.

78 "Bellevue House, Kingston." Lindy Mechefske.

83 "Hugh John Macdonald" by William Sawyer, 1852. Library and Archives Canada, e010935248.

94 "Newspaper notice of Isabella Macdonald's death and funeral." Library and Archives Canada, e008295376.

96 "Queen Victoria" by Alexander Bassano, 1882. Queen Victoria by Alexander Bassano, 1887. National Portrait Gallery London, England, x8753.

109 "A Picnic at Sloats's Lake; near Sydenham, Township of Loughborough, 1861," by Thomas Burrowes. Ref. Code: C 1-0-0-0-94 Image No.: I0002213. Archives of Ontario.

124 "The Fathers of Confederation at the London Conference." Library and Archives Canada, c006799.

133 "Susan Agnes Bernard Macdonald, 1868," by William James Topley. Library and Archives Canada, a026285.

146 "Lady Agnes Macdonald with daughter Mary, June 1869," by William James Topley. Library and Archives Canada, a033465.

156 "Drawing Room at Earnscliffe—Table set for tea." Library and Archives Canada, c006341.

165 "Label for Tomato Chutnee." Library and Archives Canada, e011081141.

168 "Russell House ca. 1893" by William James Topley. Library and Archives Canada, a008434.

181 "Old Guard Dinner 1882" by William James Topley. Library and Archives Canada, a009068.

189 "Menu and toasts booklet for banquet in honour of Sir John A. Macdonald hosted by the Liberal Conservative Party of Ontario." (detail) Library and Archives Canada, e008295515-16.

193 "Sir John A. and Lady Macdonald at a whistle-stop in Port Arthur, Ontario—September 3, 1886." Used with permission of Canadian Pacific Archives. Image No. A.18965.

199 "Sir John A. Macdonald's funeral procession on Parliament Hill, Ottawa, June 1891." Library and Archives Canada, c007125.

Bibliography

SIR JOHN A. MACDONALD AND HIS FAMILY

Angus, Margaret. *John A. Lived Here*. Kingston, ON: Frontenac History Foundation, 1984.

Biggar, Emerson Bristol. *Anecdotal Life of Sir John Macdonald*. Montreal: Lovell, 1891. https://archive.org/details/cihm_00133.

Bolger, Rev. Francis W.P. "The Charlottetown Conference and its Significance in Canadian History." *Canadian Catholic Historical Association Report*, 27, 1960.

Brown, Jacqueline A. *Sir John A. Macdonald: The Rascal Who Built Canada*. Toronto: JackFruit Press, 2005.

Bunting, Jennifer. *Sir John A's Napanee*. Kingston ON: Cranberry Hill, 1999.

Creighton, Donald. *John A. Macdonald: The Young Politician, The Old Chieftain*. Toronto: University of Toronto Press, 1998.

Gwyn, Richard. "Canada's First Scapegoat." *The Walrus*, December 2014.

———. *John A: The Man Who Made Us*. Toronto: Random House, 2008.

———. *Nation Maker: Sir John A. Macdonald: His Life, Our Times, Volume Two, 1867–1891*. Toronto: Random House, 2011.

———. "Sir John A. Macdonald made mistakes, but he wasn't a racist." *Toronto Star*, February 6, 2014.

Hammond, M.O. *Confederation and Its Leaders*. Toronto: McClelland, Goodchild & Stewart, 1917.

Hawksley, Lucinda. *The Mystery of Princess Louise: Queen Victoria's Rebellious Daughter*. London: Random House, 2013.

Johnson, J.K., ed. *Affectionately Yours: The Letters of Sir John A. Macdonald and his family*. Toronto: Macmillan of Canada, 1969.

Macpherson, James Pennington. *The Life of the Rt. Hon. Sir John A. Macdonald*. Saint John, NB: Earle Publishing House, 1891.

Martin, Ged. "John A. Macdonald and the Bottle," *Journal of Canadian Studies* 40, no. 3 (2006): 162-85.

———. *John A. Macdonald: Canada's First Prime Minister*. Toronto: Dundurn Press, 2013.

———. "Sir John Eh? Macdonald: Recovering a Voice From History." *British Journal of Canadian Studies* 17 (2004): 117-124.

McSherry, James. "The Invisible Lady: Sir John A. Macdonald's First Wife." *Canadian Bulletin of Medical History* 1, no. 1 (1984): 91-97.

Phenix, Patricia. *Private Demons: The Tragic Personal Life of John A. Macdonald.* Toronto: McClelland & Stewart, 2006.

Pope, Joseph. *Memoirs of the Right Honourable Sir John Alexander Macdonald, G.C.B., First Prime Minister of the Dominion of Canada*, vols. 1 & 2. Ottawa: J. Durie & Son, 1894. https://archive.org/details/cihm_12085.

Reynolds, Louise. *Agnes: The Biography of Lady Macdonald.* Ottawa: Carleton University Press, 1990.

Smith, Cynthia M, and Jack McLeod, eds. *Sir John A.: An Anecdotal Life of John A. Macdonald.* Don Mills, ON: Oxford University Press, 1989.

Stauffer, Rev. Byron H. "Sir John A. Macdonald, Empire Builder," *The Empire Club of Canada Addresses*, February 18, 1915.

Waite, P.B. *The Charlottetown Conference 1864*. Ottawa: Canadian Historical Association, 1970. Accessible online at Library and Archives Canada.

———. *John A. Macdonald.* Don Mills, ON: Fitzhenry & Whiteside Limited, 1976.

———. *Macdonald: His Life and World.* Toronto: McGraw-Hill Ryerson Limited, 1975.

HISTORICAL AND CONTEXTUAL REFERENCES

Canadian Pacific Railway, Canadian Pacific Railway Dining Car Service: Standard of Portions, Prices and Table Service, CPR, 1920.

Conrad, Margaret and Alvin Finkel. *History of the Canadian Peoples, 1867–Present*, vol. 2 (4th ed.) Don Mills, ON: Pearson Education Canada, 2005.

Daschuk, James William. *Clearing the Plains: Disease, Politics of Starvation, and the Loss of Aboriginal Life.* Regina, SK: University of Regina Press, 2013.

Foster, Jane. *Bath, on the Bay of Quinte*. Napanee, ON: Lennox and Addington County Museum, 1996.

Langton, Hugh Hornby, ed. *A Gentlewoman in Upper Canada: The Journals, Letters and Art of Anne Langton*. Toronto: Clarke, Irwin & Company Limited, 1950.

Moodie, Susanna. *Roughing it in the Bush: or, Life in Canada*. London: Richard Bentley, 1852.

Pope, Maurice, ed. *Public Servant: The Memoirs of Sir Joseph Pope*. Toronto: Oxford University Press, 1960.

Traill, Catharine Parr. *Female Emigrant's Guide and Hints on Canadian Housekeeping.* Toronto: MacLear and Company, 1854.

———. *The Backwoods of Canada: Being letters from the wife of an emigrant officer: Illustrative of the domestic economy of British America.* London: C. Knight, 1836.

FOOD, RECIPE, AND COOKERY BOOKS

Amis, Kingsley. *Everyday Drinking: The Distilled Kingsley Amis.* New York: Bloomsbury Publishing, 2010.

Anonymous: Compiled by The Ladies of Toronto and Chief Cities and Towns in Canada. *The Canadian Home Cook Book.* Toronto: Hunter, Rose and Company, 1877. Facsimile Edition reprinted by Coles Publishing Company, Toronto, 1971.

Anonymous. *The Canadian Housewife's Manual of Cookery: Carefully Compiled from the Best English, French & American Works, Especially Adapted to this Country.* Hamilton, ON: William Gillespy, Henry L. Richards, 1861.

Anonymous. *The Cook Not Mad; Or Rational Cookery.* Kingston, Upper Canada: James Macfarlane, 1831. Bicentennial Edition reprinted by Cherry Tree Press, Toronto, 1984. Online version available at Library and Archives Canada: http://www.collectionscanada.gc.ca/cuisine/027006-1250-e.html

Bates, Christina. *Out of Old Ontario Kitchens: A Collection of Traditional Recipes of Ontario and the Stories of the People Who Cooked Them.* Toronto: Pagurian Press, 1978.

Beeson, Patricia. *Macdonald Was Late for Dinner.* Peterborough, ON: Broadview Press, 1993.

Beeton, Isabella. *Mrs. Beeton's Book of Household Management.* England: S.O. Beeton Publishing, 1861.

Driver, Elizabeth. *Culinary Landmarks: A Bibliography of Canadian Cookbooks, 1825-1949.* Toronto: University of Toronto Press, 2008.

Fairfield, Dora E. *Dora's Cook Book.* Toronto: Hunter Rose & Co., 1888.

Fiskin, Elizabeth Davidson. *Manuscript Cookbook, circa* 1850-1860. Toronto Reference Library.

Nourse, Elizabeth. *Modern Practical Cookery, Pastry, Confectionery, Pickling and Preserving: With a Great Variety of Useful and Economical Receipts.* Montreal: Armour & Ramsay, 1845.

OTHER SOURCES

Archives of Ontario, Toronto, ON
Bellevue House, Kingston, ON
Canadian Pacific Railway Archives, Calgary, AB
Lennox and Addington County Museum and Archives, Napanee, ON
Library and Archives Canada, Ottawa, ON
Toronto Public Library Archives, Toronto, ON

Index of Recipes

Index

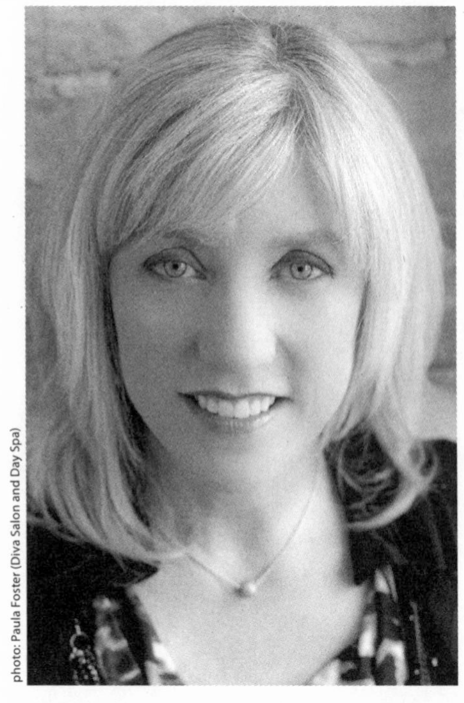

photo: Paula Foster (Diva Salon and Day Spa)

LINDY MECHEFSKE is a freelance writer and food columnist. She is the author of the cookbook *A Taste of Wintergreen* and blogs about her adventures in the kitchen at lindymechefske.com. She spent her early years in England and has lived in the USA and Australia but calls beautiful, historic Kingston, Ontario, her home. Lindy's love affairs with food and history began when she was three years old, rolling out the pastry for jam tarts in her grandfather's ancient Yorkshire kitchen.